Healing Sex

Healing Sex

A Mind–Body Approach to Healing Sexual Trauma

STACI HAINES

FELICE NEWMAN, EDITOR

CLEIS
PRESS

Published in the United States by Cleis Press Inc., P.O. Box 14697, San Francisco, California 94114.

Printed in the United States.
Cover design: Scott Idleman
Cover photograph: Getty Images
Book design: Karen Quigg
Cleis Press logo art: Juana Alicia © 1986
Illustrations copyright © 1998, 1999 by Fish.

Library of Congress Cataloging-in-Publication Data
Haines, Staci.
  Healing sex : a mind–body approach to healing sexual trauma / Staci Haines. — 2nd ed.
    p. cm.
  ISBN 978-1-57344-293-0 (alk. paper)
    1. Adult child sexual abuse victims — United States — Psychology.
2. Adult child sexual abuse victims — United States — Sexual Behavior.
3. Sex counseling — United States. 4. Sex instruction — United States.
5. Somatics I. Title
  HV6570.2.H34 2007
  362.76'4'0973—dc21   99-24107
                        CIP

Acknowledgments

I wish to thank Denise Benson for her partnership and love, and for sharing her life, children, and family with me. To Richard Strozzi-Heckler, for the generosity with which he shares his mastery and innovation in somatics. I continue to learn from him how to listen deeply to what is greater and take life-affirming action in the world. To Akaya Windwood and Maria Gonzales Baron for walking the roads of liberation together, laughing. To Jackie Strano and Shar Rednour, whose tireless efforts made the DVD *Healing Sex* possible. I appreciate your ongoing commitment to sex-positive education, images, and possibilities for people. And, lastly, to my sister, Wendy, thank you for being my family, always.

My gratitude also goes to my editor, publisher, and friend Felice Newman, without whom none of this would have happened.

Dedication

This book is dedicated to the girls that we were.
Welcome to the rest of your life, and the world you can create.
May it be filled with pleasure and wisdom.

illustrations

contents

Introduction to the Second Edition

In 1999, when this book was first published as *The Survivor's Guide to Sex: How to Have an Empowered Sex Life After Child Sexual Abuse*, I haggled over the title with the publisher. I wanted the word *somatics* in the title; the publisher understandably said no one would know what that meant. The next round continued over the term *trauma* and whether people would understand that word in the context of child sexual abuse. Now, here we are eight years later, and trauma is a more commonplace concept. Well beyond the boundaries of psychology, the general public uses the term to describe anything from the impact of war on soldiers and civilians to the intimate traumas of domestic violence and sexual abuse. And while somatics doesn't roll off of everyone's tongues, mind/body integration is recognized as something relevant to healing and learning.

There has been a profound growth in the field of trauma in the last fifteen years along with a near revolution in our understanding of the connection between psychobiology and trauma and healing. The central role of the mind/body in surviving and healing from traumatic experiences is now widely acknowledged. Somatics is the field leading these innovations, with top neurobiologists helping ground this work in studies of the brain and body chemistry before and after traumatic events.

As we head into this publication, I want to comment briefly on some of the recent research and innovations in both somatics and trauma. This new material is not included in the main body of *Healing Sex*. First, I'd like to offer a bit of science about just what is going on in our automatic survival reactions during and after traumatic experiences. Then I'll touch on the current integration of somatics into the field of psychology and what we need to be careful about as this is happening. Somatics is just now being institutionalized, and how this is done during these next years will set the course for its future. And last, I want to point to powerful innovations in looking at trauma as both an individual and a social phenomenon. This is not just the result of the obvious recent traumas of Hurricane Katrina, the tsunami in Indonesia and Asia, or the wars on Iraq and Afghanistan, but the more persistent and often unrecognized impacts of homophobia, sexism, racism, and other types of social oppression, often seen as the norm. These, too, impact us deeply.

On this last note, let me share a story. A female client of mine was struggling with her sexuality and a history of sexual abuse from her aunt. Those who have been abused by female perpetrators have an especially difficult time because this type of abuse is less talked about, and a female perpetrator contradicts our expectations and stereotypes about women. While women sexual offenders are fewer in number than men—various research shows that only 8 to 17 percent of child sexual offenders are female—women do sexually abuse. Though my client had already done a lot of healing work around her abuse, she still had little to no interest in sex with her husband and wanted to change that. Using somatics, we worked for a year on her foundational survival responses. She had little sense of what she wanted, authentically generated from her felt senses and her own values and/or calling. For many reasons, her feelings had been unacceptable and dangerous within the context of her family, and she had become good at "performing," or looking and acting how she was expected to. By the time she came to see me, these expectations were no longer necessarily those of her parents but what she thought "society" expected: this included both the social "ideals" of upward class mobility and heterosexuality. Having a reference point for her choices that was generated truly from her values, needs, and desires was what we worked to find and to build. Our fundamental impulses show up in our sensations. When we can feel ourselves deeply, we can notice what we authentically love and care about, or what we are called to. Many people experience this as both a deeply embodied (physical) and spiritual experience. For sexual trauma survivors the sheer process of being able to feel, allow, and in the best sense of the word tolerate one's own sensations is very healing. It opens the door for a self-defined, or self-referential, life. It opens the door as well to being embodied. We can see this as the antidote to dissociation.

As my client deepened into this process, what she began to reveal to herself again was her attraction to women. She had always been attracted to women and had first lived with a woman partner until they both decided that this was wrong and "supported each other" in finding male partners. Her ex retreated into fundamentalist religion, where she still resides. What we began to come up against was not the sexual abuse per se, but the impact of homophobia and how this interacted with her personal survival strategies from the abuse. If we had not begun to explore the social context we were living in (heterosexism) and its impact on her, we would have been digging in the sexual abuse without success. What we had to work with was the impact of homophobia and social oppression on her life, intimate relationships, and sexuality. She fundamentally was terrified to leave what was perceived as acceptable by society.

While the social aspect of trauma may seem obvious when talking about sexuality and sexual preference, the impact of racism, sexism, and other forms of social oppression also have a profound impact, leaving people and communities with lasting negative symptoms. So many people ask questions about who they are sexually because of the impact of prescribed sexual roles and stereotypes by religion, gender, race, and sex-negativity.

What's Happening in the Body?

Memory lives in the muscle.
—RICHARD STROZZI-HECKLER, PHD., FOUNDER OF STROZZI INSTITUTE

An easy way to think about trauma and the human brain is that the reptilian brain, the oldest part of our brains in charge of basic instincts and reproduction, and the emotional and stress centers in the brain move into overdrive. There is a high level of neuronal activity in these areas, with the corresponding release of chemicals to assist in survival. The most recently evolved part of our brains, the neocortex (frontal lobe) which also houses the speech center, is nearly shut down (showing very low levels of neuronal activity). When endangered, our brains and bodies are driven to seek safety and to protect relationships (both essential for human beings). The survival reactions are not oriented toward understanding what is happening or making sense of it at this point. Phrases like *speechless terror* are literal; certain shock and survival states show almost no neuronal activity in the brain's speech center. It is normal that people cannot control or change survival reactions to traumatic experiences by "thinking them through." To heal trauma, we must work with the parts of our brains and bodies that are mobilized for survival. What's so groundbreaking about this new understanding of the body and trauma is that it allows us to develop more relevant tools and interventions for healing.

When people are confronted with traumatic experiences, like sexual abuse, they experience an immediate physiological reaction. All animals show biologically driven responses to a threat to their own survival or, in the case of social animals, a threat to the community (pack). In humans, the instant a threat is perceived, the brain and body react, signaling the pituitary and adrenal glands to release a flood of stress hormones. These hormones—among them, adrenaline, cortisol, and norepinephrine—make survivors of trauma hyperalert, preparing them to take some kind of survival action. The fight-or-flight response is familiar to all of us. When this happens, the body gets ready to act by pumping blood into the larger "action" muscles, speeding up the heart rate, raising the blood pressure, and accelerating or holding the breath. Nonsurvival functions like hunger, sleepiness, and digestion shut down. Reproduction is also a nonsurvival function, and often this is impacted, especially through repeated trauma. Several interesting studies are being done on chronic reproductive issues for sexual abuse survivors.

When survival actions like fighting or fleeing may bring more harm or aren't viable (as is the case for many children surviving abuse), the brain and body make a third choice—the freeze response. Survivors often talk about being very still, waiting until the abuse is over, or checking out (dissociation is an inherent survival response, too). During this response, painkilling endorphins and opioids are released, and the person shifts from action to immobility. When survivors talk about not fighting back or being able to move, this is literal. Tense muscles become still, and breathing and heartbeats slow to barely perceptible. Smart, huh?

After the danger passes, our brains and bodies are designed to return to balance, or a nonhyperalert state. People often become suddenly aware that they are exhausted, hungry, or in physical pain. Our biologies inherently know how to do this. Through a process which often includes shaking and trembling, sweating, crying, and yawning, we release the increased chemicals, return the breathing to normal, relax the mobilized muscles and, if dissociated, sink back into our own skins. As we come back to a coherent, calmed state, hope is rediscovered with an overall positive orientation toward the future. When restoring balance is allowed to happen fully—and even better, when it is supported by others—there are usually few resulting symptoms of PTSD, or post-traumatic stress disorder.

The human psychobiology is oriented toward two things: survival and connection. Survival is obvious: a deep drive to be and remain alive. Connection is about being loved and loving, being accepted by the group, and being able to contribute to other people. We are social animals, and at a very biological level we orient toward connection and making meaning with others.

One thing that is so difficult about child sexual abuse and other forms of violence that are intimate is that it confuses the need to survive and the need to be connected and love. Instead of these two foundational functions operating together, they are put at odds through trauma.

In collective traumas people (because we are social animals) can often move into collective calming behaviors. It was repeatedly noted after 9/11 that New Yorkers were uncharacteristically kind to each other in public, that relations with police were warm, that there was an increase in calming physical contact. All of these behaviors are automatic and designed to calm the "collective body."

Another amazing example of collective responses to traumatic events comes from Pumla Gobodo-Madikizela, a black South African psychologist who participated in the truth and reconciliation process after the end of the apartheid regime. She noted that after political assassinations in various black townships, some townships experienced an increase in intercommunity violence and others a decrease. When studying the differences, she found that those townships that came together after

the assassinations and drummed, chanted, and danced (from a somatic perspective, calmed the collective psychobiology and made contact with the group) showed
a decrease in violence. Those townships in which people stayed more isolated and
had no collective process to work with the violation (traumatic experience) showed
increased violence. This, along with many other examples, tells us a lot about the
impact of collective traumas and some of the practices we need to be in to move
our communities toward resolving rather than perpetuating violence and trauma.

Many things prevent the natural process of discharging the hyperalert or
freeze response and returning to a calm and cohesive self or group. Often this is
prevented by a lack of knowledge of the process and the social stigmas associated
with this type of release. When, post trauma, allowing the psychobiological
process isn't viable, people override it by contracting the body even more to prevent what may seem like a strange or out-of-control emotional or physical experience. They may hold their breath and tighten the eyes and jaws so as not to cry,
contract the stomach and gut to "push the experience down," while telling themselves something like "it doesn't matter anyway" or "I'm not going to let them
get to me." An adult may tell a child, "Quit shaking, it's over, it wasn't that bad,
why are you such a scaredy-cat, anyway?" The child then has to stop what is a
natural healing process, by overriding their crying or shaking. This override prevents the healthy release and equilibrium response. Today, very few people feel
comfortable allowing themselves or supporting someone else in allowing the
release, shaking, and emoting that can return the mind/body to equilibrium after
traumatic experiences. I hope this healing process will become more socially
familiar and acceptable in the next generation.

The suppression of the release response lives on in the body as contractions
that become chronic. Many survivors of trauma report that they no longer know
how to cry or get angry. Or that whole parts of their bodies are numb or seem missing. It is not that these emotions or those parts of the body are actually gone; rather,
they have been suppressed or contracted to the point of being inaccessible. The
need to release those states, to complete a healthy response to a violation, doesn't
just go away; it gets more deeply pressed into the body and the muscles. In somatics we say that the person then begins to shape his or her self, ideas, worldview, and

actions around that experience. It is impossible not to. "Out of sight, out of mind" doesn't truly describe trauma. Rather, the traumatic experiences may be pushed out of conscious view into the more unconscious realm of the body, where the survival reactions, contractions, and somatic "shaping" continue to impact one's life.

When the body begins to thaw, or process the traumatic events, we will encounter both the contractions with which these responses were repressed as well as the incomplete responses to the trauma itself. It's as if the body's response to the original trauma has just been waiting. A somatic process includes thera-peutic conversation, somatic bodywork, and new somatic practices. Through these, we access the traumatic contractions, help them to soften, and support the psychobiological release. This in turn changes one's sense of one's self, who one is in relationship, and opens choices and new actions. Somatic practices help a survivor embody new ways to address their need for safety and connection that the survival reactions took care of. They support the mind/body to learn new ways of being and acting, rather than soley new ideas that aren't operational. Through the integral process, the inherent healing responses of the psychobiology can now be followed and supported, and new competencies embodied.

The Future of Somatics

In the West, the field of somatics harkens back to the early 1900s and Wilhelm Reich. Many other cultures have long understood the mind, body, and spirit (and often one's connection to land) as integral and important to healing and restor-ing well-being. With Descartes and others, we in the West inherited a different view, one of the mind as separate from the flesh. This central cultural and reli-gious assumption influences our understanding of the body and promotes the view of it as an object and/or shameful. The prevailing paradigm of mind over flesh also informs our cultural stereotypes about women, emotions, sexuality, and race. The more one is perceived as being connected to the flesh, or the earth, the lower one's perceived status or social value. Somatics challenges this orientation.

Somatics is now gaining more recognition after decades of development in the West and recent research in neuropsychology and trauma. Some of the most influential people who have contributed their understanding, research, and approaches to somatics in the last century include Ida Rolf, Alexander Lowen, Fritz Perls, George Leonard, Randolph Stone, Emilie Conrad, Moshé Feldenkrais, Anna Halprin, and Richard Strozzi-Heckler. The field is beginning to be institutionalized, with more universities offering degrees in somatics, particularly somatic psychology, and generalized standards are being developed. The integration of somatics into psychology makes sense, given that much of somatics is used for healing. The use of somatics in learning, leadership development, and social movements is also powerful, but fits less readily into a given mold. As this institutionalization happens, however, there are benefits and drawbacks.

First, however, let's define somatics. Its Greek root means "the living body in its wholeness." Somatics is a new interpretation of the self as well as the collective "body." It is not the body "added on" to traditional psychotherapy. It is a new paradigm, like the concept of the unconscious mind was a century ago. This new paradigm leads to new understanding, new possibilities, and new actions. Along with the view of the mind, body, and spirit as one integrated whole, some somatic approaches also integrate an understanding of the social context, land, and the collective body. Perhaps what is most unique about somatics is that it treats the body as an essential place of change, learning, and transformation. Somatics sees the "self," or who we are, as inseparable from the body. When we reconnect the vast intelligence of the body with the mind and spirit, powerful change and healing are available. The somatics discourse combines somatic awareness, somatic bodywork, and somatic practices to create lasting change.

The majority of foundational somatic training institutes are still independent of the university setting. There are a variety of quality somatic approaches. Those that are being more readily integrated into the field of psychology are "attention based" rather than hands-on somatic theories and practices. These somatic interventions attend to the sensations in the body, through conversation and cognition. By tracking sensations, the body is cultivated as a base of knowledge and change. However, essential aspects of somatics—including somatic practices and somatic bodywork—are being left out. The somatic interventions and theory that fit more readily into verbal dialogue and into therapists' training, current theoretical frameworks, and techniques are being taught instead. The full potency of somatics is in danger of being diluted.

There is a historical bias in the field of psychology *away from* the body. Simply put, the default orientation is that changing the mind, one's interpretations, and one's emotional responses lead to an individual's transformation. The body is not seen as a central player in this. Psychology also actively discourages touch, which is often associated with sex, sexual harassment, and the misuse of power within the therapeutic relationship, or inappropriate boundaries generating unnecessary complications. If one is not ethical or trained, this can certainly be the case. But, like any other set of skills, becoming competent and masterful in somatics means having strong teachers, powerful feedback, and a community with which to practice. This includes the powerful and ethical use of somatic touch. There is a lively debate within somatic psychology circles about the ethics of *not* using somatic touch when it is often the most effective and relevant tool for healing and transformation.

Somatics fundamentally invites a new set of questions into psychology based on the effectiveness of this new paradigm and the brain research to ground it. We are at an important turning point in the integration of somatics into the broader culture. We can keep its full power by integrating somatic awareness, somatic practices, and somatic touch as inseparable components of the discourse.

Social Context, Trauma, and Somatics

Since the publication of the first edition, I have been working more extensively with the social aspect of trauma and healing. Just as we see the power of integrating mind and body in healing, we also need to more deeply understand the social and political context in which we live and from whence many of our experiences of trauma rise. As in the example at the beginning of this introduction, experiences of child sexual abuse and experiences of a more systemic attack on sexuality, like homophobia, both create traumatic impact that needs healing and change. As I train therapists, healers, and practitioners in somatics and trauma work, I meet many who are wholehearted in their intent to support and help individuals transform. Yet most have not been educated in seeing the social context in which they live or their own biases. Unwittingly, therapists can perpetuate some of the same ideas and practices that cause harm, like certain concepts about gender and sexuality or racism and economic status. Without understanding more about the social systems and histories in which we live, survivors too can try to hold themselves to some version of being "normal" that may actually be harmful. As practitioners help support change in an individual's life, they can miss addressing or empowering the person to address the causes of his or her pain and suffering that are not personal, like the impact of poverty, racism, sexism, or immigration laws.

When we talk about social context, we are talking about beliefs and practices inherited through our culture and the time in history in which we live. This is like trying to see water as a fish. The region and country in which you were raised and live, your cultural identity, religious or spiritual orientation, and the organizations, economic, and governmental systems in which you operate, make up your social context. For example, a person steeped in the Catholic tradition has very different interpretations about life, the universe, meaning, and ethics than someone raised in the Buddhist tradition. Or a person who lives in a working class community has a very different set of experiences and perspective than someone who is of the owning class. This is true for all of us, and it is unavoidable. We can, however, learn to have some perspective on our own assumptions and see our own social context more clearly. Why is this important? Our unexamined assumptions have unintended consequences. This is as true in healing and social change work as in economic and government policy.

Let me give you a personal example. I was raised in the United States, in a white, working-class family of Irish, German, and other unknown northern European decent. I learned that an individual, although a part of a family, was the central identity. I heard, over and over, "Pick yourself up by your bootstraps"; "Nobody's fault but your own"; "You can be whatever you want if you work hard enough"; "It is all up to you." The collective was important, but it was not what made up your identity. For many, many other peoples and cultures, however, this is not the case. In fact, individualism is a fairly recent invention in human history.

In my practice I was working with a man who was from a culture and country in which the collective was the central way to understand the world. The idea of the individual as a separate, sovereign entity was not present in his community's worldview. He experienced sexual abuse within his broader family, as well as many traumatic experiences related to racism and immigration to the United States. Many assumptions of Western healing approaches were irrelevant to him. Western psychology is based on the assumption of the individual as the site of change and the person as singular. Family systems therapy steps out of this to some extent in that the family becomes the site of change, but the orientation of individualism still runs deep. In our work together, we had to change most of the exercises and interventions to orient toward an understanding of the person as inseparable from the collective. Instead of healing an individual, or setting boundaries with someone's abusive behavior, we needed to work with bringing healing to the whole collective body and cleansing an energy or entity that was harming all of them. This then tapped immediately into violations his people had experienced through civil wars and colonization.

When examining the biases in our own worldviews, we need to look at the benefits and costs of what we have inherited. Individualism has implications; it opens some choices and limits others. If we project it as the norm, then we are acting as oppressors. If we do not learn to begin to see, assess, and critique some of our assumptions, our actions may not reflect what we care about or mean. We may perpetuate problems or systems that we actually want to heal and change. Unfortunately, in today's psychotherapeutic tradition, learning to see our own inherited social and cultural biases is not often taught. Practitioners need to search this out through other types of education. See the Resources under *Social Trauma* for some places to start.

Much work by indigenous and third world scholars, researchers, and practitioners is about historical trauma and the collective ongoing impact of histories of colonization or slavery. These theories and approaches talk about the ongoing traumatic impact on those who were colonized and their cultures as well as on the colonizers and their lineages as well.

Somatics looks at the deep collective impact of disembodiment within many Western traditions, and the implications in many religious traditions of holding the body as shameful. These beliefs and practices disconnect us from our felt, lived experiences and have an impact on our ability to feel interconnected with other life and the earth or be empathetic with others. From a dissociated state, one in which there is decreased feeling, it is much easier to objectify others. From objectification, commodifying people and the earth, and dominating them follow. While this demands a much more comprehensive analysis than what we have room for here, I want to nod to the connections.

When I was getting my B.A. at Oberlin College, I began very reluctantly—really, kicking and screaming—to deal with my own history of child sexual abuse. I went to Student Psychological Services and asked them if they had a group for incest survivors that I could join. They told me that child sexual abuse was a rare experience and that they didn't really have someone who worked with this. But, they went on, if I could gather a group of eight survivors of child sexual abuse, they could facilitate a group for me. So there I was, depressed and desperate, my world falling apart, organizing the first survivor's group on campus. I put up flyers, ran information in the college paper, distributed my information for folks to contact me, and started talking it up on campus. I had to go public in order to get help. Within two weeks I had ten people. I went back to Psych Services. They were surprised, but they started the group. The stir of conversations on this small campus about sexual abuse led to discussions about campus rape and sexual assault, and another group emerged. This one took on campus organizing against sexual assault, trying to change the college policies and practices, and doing general consciousness-raising and prevention work.

This experience reflected something that took me much longer to articulate, although I felt it deeply…that personal transformation and social transformation are inherently connected. I see this both from the perspective of individual healing being empowered by understanding a longer history of social change work, and social movements being empowered by personal transformation. We want to eliminate the causes of the harm, not just help an endless stream of people or communities heal from trauma. In the case of child sexual abuse we might ask questions like: What creates offenders? How do we change those factors? Why are sex, ownership, and violation so connected in our culture, and how can we change that? Through social change work, we can facilitate both individual healing and preventing others from being violated in the first place.

About Me

For the last ten years I have been involved in building generation FIVE, a national nonprofit organization whose mission is to end the sexual abuse of children within five generations. This has been another way to take what is hidden public and to mobilize others into positive action for change and healing. For me, generation FIVE has also been a place to explore and invent ways to connect personal change and social change. Through a national collaborative we have developed a transformative justice approach to address child sexual abuse and other forms of intimate and community violence. The aim of transformative justice is to help secure survivor safety, support, and agency; offender accountability and recovery, and engage the broader community in prevention and social change. This approach is designed to respond to incidences of child sexual abuse in ways that are in line with long-term prevention. Child sexual abuse does not happen in a vacuum; it is a social issue requiring collective action. For more information about transformative justice, please see generation FIVE's Web site at www.generationFIVE.org.

I am still in my own process of growth and being with my own history of sexual abuse and trauma. It is not forefront in my personal work and development anymore, yet it is and always will be a part of me. Within the last year my family of origin met for the graduation of one of my nephews. My family has sadly organized itself into "camps" related to the sexual abuse, and this was the first time in fifteen-plus years that the whole crew came together. I was surprised by the relief I felt at having everyone in one place. Polarization takes energy, and I had the opportunity to let go of that, if only briefly. Sadly, the "reunion" did little to advance the healing of our family.

My family, like many others, tried to deal with familial and community sexual abuse on its own. I did not know then to organize allies for myself, people to help educate and guide the bystanders in our family and community, or to find people influential in my father's life to encourage and insist upon his accountability as well as his humanity. Because so often we see healing as individual, the importance of developing allies is many times missed. I did seek healing and therapy, and after exploring the consequences of a legal approach, I did not want to go there. In general, however, therapy focuses on the individual and not the entire dynamic of abuse and long-term change for the collective. The vision for safety, accountability, and reconciliation was mine alone to hold and try to figure out how to accomplish. In my family's case, it hasn't worked.

One thing I walked out of the reunion with, along with my outrage being rekindled, was the palpable remembering of the sheer waste of child sexual abuse for everyone. This experience also knocked out a sense of remaining hope I had had. People make choices, and these choices have real consequences. I can imagine that admitting to sexually abusing your own children and then facing the process of accountability and reconciliation may be one of the most difficult things a person could do. Yet, without it, what possibility is there of transformation or authentic relationship?

I have heard many sexual trauma survivors talk about choosing the road of optimism or the road of pessimism. If I look through that lens, I chose the former. What has been sobering, at times enraging, and fundamentally had me grieve the next level of loss…is really looking at what is and isn't happening in my family, without filling in the empty and difficult places with my optimism. Just looking at what is, and the many choices made and not made these last twenty years.

This experience was a reminder for me that the road through the center is the road that grants freedom. It isn't that it is not painful or there is not suffering. It isn't that, in my version, filling in with optimism wasn't helpful. But facing what is, albeit more painful in the short run, is ultimately more freeing, more healing. Turning and facing pain isn't the easy road, but it offers a sense of dignity and of power. It opens our futures to more choices and more possibilities of compassion and action in the world.

Staci Haines
San Francisco
August 2007

Introduction

A Personal Journey

Healing Sex confronts a double taboo: women's sexuality and child abuse, both subjects our culture would rather have us whisper about behind closed doors or, better yet, deny entirely. Yet for survivors, sex was the very site of attack. Children can be abused verbally, emotionally, physically, and through many forms of neglect. Why, then, *sexual* abuse? Why were we wounded in our most intimate places? I believe that sexual assault is an attempt to disempower, own, or destroy another. Alice Miller calls childhood sexual abuse "soul murder." Many survivors would agree with her. I often felt that my perpetrators were reaching for my soul, trying to take something from me that was long lost in themselves.

Women's sexuality is the other piece of the double taboo. What is so threatening about a sexually empowered woman? A sexually empowered woman is a woman who is embodied, whose sexual expression is a part of herself, and whose sex life is self-defined. A sexually empowered woman is able to make choices for herself; she is able to express consent and maintain boundaries that serve her. She can ask for what she wants. She becomes self-referential, meaning she trusts her own experience and intelligence over external messages. Incest is the ultimate training in not trusting one's self. Becoming sexually empowered restores that self-trust.

The wounds of children victimized by sexual abuse are so profoundly deep that most of us find ourselves turning away in denial or blaming the victims themselves. Yet one in three girls, and one in six boys, are victims of childhood sexual abuse. Few of us can face this cultural dis-ease. Whom might you see if you looked? Someone in your own family? Your favorite soccer coach, your child's music teacher, or your next-door neighbor?

I came to sex education and sexual healing through a very personal route. As is true for many women, my own healing began while I was having sex with a boyfriend. This was my moment of clarity, when I faced the fact that I had been sexually abused by my father and several "family friends" for much of my youth. I had no idea what was going on—I only knew that some internal boulder had rolled away from the mouth of the cave, and my history came pouring out.

Thus my healing journey began. I spent two years running from recovery before I finally surrendered to my healing. Before I finally faced the abuse, I experienced insomnia, an inability to eat, and a thick brick wall of depression that separated me from the world. The years that followed were horrible and miraculous. I found healing, devastation, loss, confrontation, a family falling apart and weaving (partly) together again. If you are healing from childhood sexual assault, you know exactly what I am talking about. You have stories of your own.

During the years of abuse, my survival depended upon a strong spiritual connection, a natural talent for dissociating, and being a high achiever. When I began studying the effects of trauma on children's lives, I found that survivors usually fall into the under- or overachiever camps. We are the really good kids or the really bad kids. Discovering this was a relief for me. As is true for many survivors, no one ever asked me what was up, because I was doing so well.

Actually, my second-grade teacher did ask me why I was going to the bathroom so frequently. I had chronic vaginal and yeast infections. I didn't know what was causing the itching and pain, so I would go to the bathroom a lot to check. Eventually, she pulled me aside and asked what was going on. When I didn't say anything, she asked me to go home and talk with my mom about what was happening. That was the wrong place to turn for help. Ashamed, I told my mom over dinner. She said it was just discharge and that all the women in our family had it (which speaks volumes about my family).

By junior high I was a master at dissociation. I would sit in science class and stare at my own arm. It seemed utterly bizarre to me that this was my arm. How could it be my arm? What was my arm, anyway? Except for athletics—where it was safe to feel my physical self—I did not relate to being *in* my body.

My tactic was to control my emotions and feelings, including sexual ones. In high school, I couldn't comprehend the whole "blue balls" thing the boys complained about. I could turn my sexual interest on and off again, easy as that. I wondered why others couldn't do that, too. As a kid, I didn't masturbate, and neighborhood games of truth-or-dare brought on huge attacks of shame if they involved anything even remotely sexual.

While I controlled my sexual feelings and desire, my sister's survival tactics were the opposite. Instead of controlling sex, she was out exploring with all the neighborhood kids. She says she was considered very sophisticated about sex in our neighborhood.

Once I began having consensual sex in high school, I organized my intimate life in the classic survivor split: My best friend was a guy with whom I shared my emotional life, my secrets, and my philosophical reflections. My boyfriend, with whom I explored sex, was someone else. I could hardly speak a word to him. I actually did love him but was terrified to share myself with him. I could not endure emotional intimacy and sex at the same time. I froze.

I was uninterested in other girls, who seemed weak and sissy-like to me. I hated pink. All my friends were boys. I didn't want to be a man, but I certainly was not going to be a woman. I identified as androgynous. It wasn't until I was exposed to feminism in college, and discovered powerful female role models, that I began calling myself a woman.

Somatic Healing

Much of my healing took place while I was a student at Oberlin College. It was a gift to find myself in the center of such a politicized and socially aware community. I knew that I was not alone in surviving abuse. When I couldn't heal for myself, I healed to make a difference for the future. Brave women before me had survived sexual assault and had made my life easier by their choices. I wanted to be a part of that chain of hope for others. Having that larger social context in which to see my abuse was very empowering. I organized the first incest survivors' group on campus and formed a student activist group to deal with the college's inadequate response to rape on campus. I advocated for government financial support for incest survivors and won grants to fund survivors' recovery resources.

Early on in recovery, I worked with someone who practiced body-oriented therapy. I am so grateful to her. She helped me work the trauma out of my body and opened my emotional life to me again.

The abuse seemed to pour out of my body. The more I reconnected with my body, the clearer I became about what trauma was stored where. My thighs retained rage. Moving my thighs and kicking my legs allowed me to begin expressing my anger. My chest held much of the deep grief. Where my body had been pinned or frozen during the abuse, I now began to move. How many times had I wanted to push someone off of me and couldn't? I learned how to let my arms and body do that. The relief was incredible. The process was painful. I was coming back to me. I started to identify my body not only as a shell that housed my "self" but as a source of wisdom and inspiration. My body actually knew things about the healing process that I didn't. In the thawing out, I got to live inside myself again.

Since then, I've learned that the somatic processes I went through are consistent with processes of survivors of all forms of trauma. War veterans, Holocaust survivors, and even victims of severe auto accidents experience similar processes of dissociation and freezing or holding in the body. The somatic release of these holdings allows us to process and complete trauma.

Through the healing, my sexuality emerged from a new place in me. It became less and less about how sex was supposed to look and more about my own experience of sex and desire. I had been quite sexually active during my two years of running from the healing process, but I could not really be present while having sex. I was going ninety miles an hour in my own head. I didn't know how to say what I wanted and didn't really know I had permission to do so. As I healed, this changed. My own sexual interests and preferences emerged from beneath the incest. I began to date women—and I have been sexual with women since then. The more the trauma poured out of me, the more I filled *me* in.

As may be the case for you, sex triggered me. I would be having a fine time and suddenly find myself feeling afraid, used, and abused. As I got turned on, images of the abuse appeared; it became impossible to separate *then* from *now*. My sexual response had become intermingled with abuse and betrayal. So when I experienced one, the other followed. Untangling these became my project. I would make lists to differentiate them: "What is sex?" "What is abuse?"

I slowly learned to keep myself present, allowing myself to practice sexual turn-ons that were connected to *my* body and *my* pleasure. I felt a lot of shame and guilt. *Am I allowed pleasure? If I like sex now, does it mean I wanted the abuse? Can I be the one who says what kind of touch and sex I want?* I continued to release the trauma from my body. What was caught in me that I wanted to express? How could I live deeply inside of me? As I healed, it dawned on me that sexual energy was a positive and powerful force in my own recovery.

Good Vibrations

From 1991 to 1995, I worked at Good Vibrations, the "clean well-lighted place for sex toys." Joanie Blank founded Good Vibrations in 1977 to provide a place for women to purchase sex toys and have access to positive and accurate information about sex and their own sexuality. Her small one-room retail space with a staff of three has grown into two retail stores, a Web site and mail-order operation, and a workforce that can barely fit into the staff photo in the front of the catalog. Moreover, Good Vibrations has become a leader in the field of sex education.

This was a great experience for me as a survivor of childhood sexual abuse, albeit challenging and triggering at times. Through my experience and training at Good Vibrations, I learned more about sex than I even knew I wanted to know. Where incest had taught me the most destructive uses of sex, here I sat amid a plethora of sex-positive information. Sex became normalized for me. All of this sex-positivity balanced the scales. Now I knew both the worst and the best of sex.

As a manager at Good Vibrations, however, I found myself caught repeatedly between two worlds: the world of survivors, hurt and at times paranoid about sex, and the world of sex-positive educators, many of whom did not want to hear about the negative uses of sex or the effects of sexual abuse.

Many in the survivors' community were afraid of sex and thought the best they could hope for would be something slightly better than just tolerating it. Survivors who liked sex and who spoke openly about it were met with mistrust and even, at times, disdain. It was assumed that they were "acting out" their sexual abuse. Pleasure was suspect. To me, it seemed to boil down to no trust in sex. Understandable, but not the recovery I hoped for.

Among sex educators, there was little talk of sexual violence or the sexual contradictions experienced by women who have been sexually violated. In a culture where sex is simultaneously vilified and used to sell you everything you can think of, confusion and negativity about sex is rampant. The call to sex-positivity and women's sexual self-definition was welcome. Still, I found myself educating the educators about the effects of childhood sexual abuse on adult sexuality. One colleague went so far as to suggest that incest itself wasn't the problem, that it was the cultural taboo surrounding incest that was harmful. *No, no, no!*

Educating the Educators

So I became a bridge, talking about sex with survivors and professionals who worked with them, and talking about childhood sexual abuse with sex-positive sex educators. To me, sexual empowerment seemed a normal outgrowth of healing childhood sexual abuse, and working to end the sexual abuse of children an obvious banner for the sex-positive community to fly.

I found myself longing for a place where I could talk about all of it: sex, sexual abuse, rape and its effects on sex, and the glory and healing powers of consensual adult sexuality and embodiment. I wanted to have conversations that went further than the ABCs of childhood sexual abuse ("Yes, it really does happen, and yes, it really does hurt the child, and yes, most often the abuser is someone close to the child") or the ABCs of sex education ("Yes, sex really is a natural part of being human, and yes, there are words for 'down there,' and yes, you are allowed to ask for what you want sexually"). The opportunity came when *On Our Backs* magazine asked me to write a series of articles in 1995. Felice Newman, co-publisher of Cleis Press, read my first article and called me. Thus, the beginning of this book.

Healing Sex is written for women survivors of childhood sexual abuse. Male survivors of abuse will find the tools and resources useful for their recovery as well. Survivors and non-survivors alike will find the embodiment approach to sexual recovery a refreshing antidote to the sex-negativity of our culture.

A Path Through the Wreckage

Miraculously, most survivors want to find a path through the wreckage of sexual trauma to sexual enjoyment. And why not? Sex is a fundamental human drive, one that brings pleasure, delight, ease, connection, and embodiment into our lives. I see sexual healing as the cornerstone of empowerment for the hundreds and thousands of us who have been sexually molested as children. For most survivors to allow pleasure, much less embodied sexual pleasure, into their lives is a feat. Once you begin to reclaim and re-embody sexually, you can enter the place of trauma and relinquish its control over you. You can bring peace and vitality back into your life.

At a recent International Conference on Somatics, Emilie Conrad, the founder of Continuum, a somatic approach, said, "The more you are in your own experience, sensations, your own body, the less some external or authoritarian system can control you."

Behind this book is a vision of ending the sexual abuse of children and building a world that it welcoming, safe, and respectful of their humanity. Embodiment and the power of reclaiming your own sexuality are both a part of this societal healing. People who are embodied—not dissociated nor anesthetized—are much less likely to abuse children or stand by while others abuse them.

As a somatics practitioner, I have watched survivors return to the sensations and intelligence of their bodies as a place of healing. This book is filled with information, suggestions, and exercises to help you reoccupy your body. Waking up somatically will make you more aware of yourself and your surroundings. You will become a more powerful contributor to your family, your community, and the world.

I see sexual healing as the cornerstone of empowerment for the hundreds and thousands of us who have been sexually molested as children. For most survivors to allow pleasure, much less embodied sexual pleasure, into their lives is a feat. Once you begin to reclaim and re-embody sexually, you can take back the very ground of attack. You are returning to the center of a war zone and declaring the territory yours. You get to own your life.

I see our capacity to recover as extraordinary. I have met so many survivors—close friends, somatics clients, the women who are quoted in this book—who have been resilient through extreme abuse. The more stories I hear, the more I am stunned by the extent of the sexual abuse of children and the more I am awed be the regenerative power of our spirits and humanity.

If you are a survivor of childhood sexual abuse ready to begin this journey, congratulations! I hope that this book brings you healing along with pleasure, hope, and laughter. I wish you a satisfying, embodied sex life, a life that is your own lovely creation. You are more powerful than what happened to you.

San Francisco
May 1999

chapter one

Safety, Somatics, and Sexual Healing

The Choice to Heal

Is your sexuality a healthy and integrated part of you? Can you talk easily about sex, your sexual desires, and your sexual healing and needs? Are you able to know and communicate your sexual boundaries?

These are admittedly leading questions. Many survivors do not have a good reference point for their own sexual well-being and pleasure. And why should you? Childhood sexual abuse is not what you might call positive input about sex or your own sexuality. To begin this process of sexual recovery it is vital to know *why* you want to embark on this journey. What do you want to gain from healing sexually? How do you want your sex life to be different?

> *It took me a long time to decide to heal sexually. I kept thinking, "Why go through all of that? Sex, I can take it or leave it." But something kept tugging at me, like a part of me wanted to be whole again.*—Hannah

Motivations for Healing

So why heal sexually, anyway? What do you want in your sex life that you do not have now? What would it be like to not find triggers around every corner? To fully experience sexual pleasure and expression? Ask yourself these questions.

What motivated me initially is that I couldn't say "no." I was having sex with people I did not want to have sex with, looking for attention and acknowledgment through sex. At first I just wanted and needed to stop doing this; then, slowly it began to dawn on me that I could actually have sex based on what I wanted and needed. That I could have sex that I liked.—Kathy

Some motivations for healing will sustain you through the process better than others. Deciding to heal because you think you are "bad" or "dirty" or believe something is "wrong" with you won't necessarily serve your cause. Most folks eventually tune out negative motivations —or rebel against them. Developing a positive motivation is more sustaining and will give you a vision to work toward. If you are unable to think of positive motivations, ask a friend or support person to help you brainstorm at least three positive reasons to heal sexually. Many survivors want to heal to save their relationship or please their partner. Perhaps your partner wants to have sex but you don't. While sex *is* an important part of any intimate partnership, you need to develop motivations that are just for you. Pressure from a partner can make it

> ### *Positive Motivations for Sexual Healing*
>
> • I want to gain a freedom in my body. I want to be able to move, make noise, and express myself fully.
>
> • I want to heal the shame that runs my sex life so that I feel relaxed and excited during sex.
>
> • I want to enjoy touching myself.
>
> • I want my body back, all the way.
>
> • I want pleasure and being present in my sex life to be the norm, instead of fear and checking out.
>
> • I want to have sex in the ways I am interested in. I want to be more courageous sexually.
>
> • I want to be able to respect and communicate my sexual boundaries.
>
> • I want to learn that I am loved for me and not for sex alone.
>
> • I want to be make my own sexual choices.
>
> • I want to have sex and intimacy at the same time.

difficult to tell whether you are really making a choice. Encouragement is wonderful, but you still have to want to do this work. You will not speed up the healing process by having sex that is forced, dissociated, or checked out.

I didn't want him to leave me. He had been so good through this whole mess, I just wanted to please him. The sex wasn't even good when I just did it for him, but at least I was giving him sex, I thought. I couldn't "heal" just to make him stay, though. It was only when I tuned into how my life could be different, how I might feel more positively about myself, that I made any progress in sex.—Sheila

Last, you do not need to have a sexual partner to be actively sexual. Nor does sexual healing have to wait for a lover. The concepts and exercises outlined in this book apply to you whether you are partnered or single. Many people do much of their sexual healing work on their own and then move into a relationship with new tools and knowledge.

The decision to heal sexually is a choice to reclaim an aspect of yourself that has been wounded and used. It is a choice to make whole again a very powerful and vital aspect of your being. This process can be extremely uncomfortable, yet it can give you amazing freedom, pleasure, and satisfaction. It can give you *you* back.

Safety and Sexual Healing

Safety is an odd concept for most survivors of childhood sexual abuse. I'm usually met with raised eyebrows when I ask survivors about feeling safe and being sexual. Incest and childhood sexual abuse are frightening experiences that undermine the development of your sense of safety in yourself, your body, your relationships, your sexuality, and the world.

When it comes to sex, I am terrified. People talk about safety, and I can't relate to that. Feeling safe and having sex seem to live in two separate worlds.
—Carla

Safety is complicated for survivors. During the abuse your safety was out of your hands. If you could have done anything to make it stop, you would have. Really. The intelligent mistake you, like most survivors, probably made as a kid was thinking that you had some control over your safety. You didn't. Children are manipulated, coerced, threatened, and forced into sexual abuse, sometimes under the guise of love.

I thought if I could just be good enough, smart enough, nice enough, perfect enough that I could keep me and my brother safe. It never worked. I never succeeded. I am not really sure what else to do to be safe.—Rona

What's tricky is that now you need to develop a sense of safety to move into your sexual healing. Without a sense of safety, you cannot engage your sexuality. You especially can't take on new challenges and growth if you don't feel safe. How do you know when you are safe?

What Is Safety?

Most people think of safety as a "feeling" of being safe. While this is one way to judge safety, it is not always reliable. You can be in a very safe situation and feel unsafe because you are dealing with an aspect of your abuse. Or, because you are a trauma survivor, you may be in an unsafe situation and feel just fine. While feeling safe is important, it does not necessarily give you reliable ground upon which to determine if you are safe, or safe enough to proceed.

WHAT TELLS YOU THAT YOU ARE SAFE?

When checking in on your safety in a given situation, consider the following:

- How do you feel in your body? Do you feel safe, scared, unsettled?
- Is your physical environment safe and free of violence and abuse? (No one is hitting, kicking, punching, or pushing you. No one is calling you names or threatening you or anyone you care about.)
- Does your partner, lover, or friend consider your needs, wants, and desires as important and relevant as his or her own?
- Can your partner, lover, or friend really meet your needs? Does he or she have the know-how, the tools, and the good intention?
- Do you have the power in this situation to act upon your own behalf? To take care of yourself fully?
- Are you making your own choices? Not being pressured, pushed, or manipulated?

Asking yourself these questions gives you a way to assess whether or not you are safe—even when you do not necessarily feel safe.

Being safe and feeling comfortable are not the same thing. You might be able to answer the above questions in a way that lets you know you are safe, but still find that you feel afraid and uncomfortable. Sexual healing does not always feel safe; in fact, it can feel downright scary.

While you didn't have power as a child to act on your own behalf and take care of yourself, you do now. You get to decide whether or not a situation is safe for you and then decide what to do about it. When you are safe, you are able to make your own choices. You are empowered to take care of yourself.

Building a Sense of Internal Safety

When you have had little sense of true safety in your life, how do you go about building some? Once your external safety has been handled, safety becomes an inside job. You can develop a sense of internal safety, a way of feeling in your body that lets you know you are okay and that everything is all right. This ability to relax or let down your guard is often what was so damaged through sexual abuse. Even when your relationships and the world you have built around you are safe, you may feel like you are never really safe. Most trauma survivors experience this feeling of low-level, insistent, persistent danger.

> Mentally I know that I am safe now. I mean, stuff happens in the world, I may get shot or raped. But given that I am in a safe home and safe relationships and have taken self-defense, my odds even of that are low. So why is it that I feel I am always watching on some level? If I come off guard, I think that will be the moment they have been waiting for to attack me. I'd rather get attacked when I have my defenses up. I don't think I could bear trusting again and being attacked when I am relaxed.—Maggie

To build an internal sense of safety, let's look to your body. What sensations do you feel there? Notice temperature, pressure, and movement. Notice sensation all over your body, front and back, inside and out, top and bottom. Do you feel warmth in your legs? Cool feet? Tension in your stomach? Tingling inside your head? Are you feeling blocked or rigid in your chest?

Now, look for a place in your body where you feel a sense of peace, strength, or well-being. Do you feel strength in the palms of your hands? A sense of well-being in your right hip? Where do you feel your body comfortably settling? A sense of openness or spaciousness? Look for the literal sensations. What are they?

If you are unable to find a place in your body where you experience comfort, find something you like outside of your body. Think of your favorite animal, a beautiful color, a person you love, a place in nature, or something you love to do, like singing, skiing, or surfing. Notice what happens in your body. Does a smile come across your face? A feeling of warmth spread across your chest or back? Maybe your hips relax and get warm. These sensations are the building blocks for your sense of internal well-being. You can call these your sensations of safety or pleasure, well-being, or resourcefulness. These are what we will use in building a strong internalized sense of safety.

Bring your attention back to these sensations again. Have they changed at all? Sensations in the body are alive and shifting all the time. Place your attention on your body and look openly at where you feel those resourceful sensations now. What are those sensations like? Are they moving?

Now practice making those sensations smaller. Can you shrink them down? And bigger. Can you expand that warmth or spaciousness? What is it like to sit and breathe with these resourceful sensations for thirty seconds? Try this now. I will ask you throughout the book to call forth these sensations of safety. The more you notice them, the more apparent and present they will become. Noticing these sensations does not make other sensations, feelings of fear and anger, or triggers go away; rather, it gives you a safe place to approach them from. By accessing these sensations again and again, you can build an internalized sense of safety or resourcefulness to return to when facing challenging moments in your healing—or even when you are having sex.

What's Down This Road, Anyway?

Your sexual healing process will be affected by many factors, including the particular abuse you experienced, who the perpetrators were, and the quality of support available to you then and now. The information or misinformation you have received about sex will also come into play. Your cultural, class, and religious background will help frame the uniqueness of your journey. If you were raised Catholic, you will have a different set of issues to grapple with than someone raised in a non-religious household. Your experiences of social bias and oppression add to the mix.

The pain and uncertainty of incest felt very much like the insecurities of being a person of color, a woman, and gay in this culture. The result is disempowerment.—Lee

Expect to experience a gamut of emotions. Terror, rage, grief, and guilt will have their turns alongside new types of excitement, pleasure, and desire. Issues and emotions that you thought you had dealt with long ago may arise. At times you may feel like you are going backward. Do not be discouraged. This is normal in the sexual healing process. Because you are now healing the very arena in which you were abused, issues of boundaries, consent, dissociation, and triggers are necessarily a part of the work.

As I began to focus on being sexual and recovering this part of me, I found myself dealing with being afraid of people again and not being able to sit still. These seemed unrelated to my sexual healing at first, but they were just a new layer of fears to work through in being more sexual.—Jeanie

I have worked a lot on being able to stay present and not disappear, and I have made a lot of progress. The hardest part of sexual healing is dealing with how I shut down. Staying present during sex is a whole new thing.—Terri

You can think of sexual healing as graduate-level recovery.

Although I remembered my sexual abuse during sex, and remained sexually active throughout most of my process, I am seven years into my healing and just now getting into the real stuff of sex. I am now giving myself permission to really express myself sexually, learning to be in my body during sex, and getting a glimpse of what intimacy and sex combined could be like.—Danielle

Your healing process will most likely proceed at an uneven pace. You'll find there will be times of intense focus and times of rest. Sometimes you just have to attend to other aspects of your life. You'll develop a rhythm of moving into and then back out of the work of sexual healing.

Hot Spots in Healing

Along the way, you may have to grapple with some difficult contradictions. You may find that there are aspects of the abuse that were physically pleasurable to you. You may have come to orgasm during the abuse, or you may have loved the attention you received. Your perpetrators may have deliberately turned you on. You are not bad, wrong, or to blame. Sexual and sensual response is normal and healthy. Your body and sexuality did not betray you; your perpetrators did.

> *My orgasms have been very hard to come by. My abuser brought me to orgasm as part of his game. I have had to practice forgiving myself over and over again, just acknowledging that my body responded like any healthy body would.*
> *—Shandell*

You may have engaged in nonconsensual sex play with other children. Sometimes children who are being abused act out the abuse on other children or even pets. This may have been sexually arousing or erotic to you, and you may carry feelings of guilt and shame. Facing each of these experiences is part of the healing and self-forgiveness required to free yourself.

> *My family would hang out with my younger cousins in the summer. The second year my dad was abusing me, I started touching my cousins. It's like I was trying to work out on them what was happening to me.—Dede*

You may enjoy some sexual acts now that were perpetrated on you as a child and dislike others. You may be simultaneously attracted to and repulsed by certain fantasies related to your abuse. Your sexual desires, fantasies, and sexual responses are affected by the abuses you suffered as well as other personal, family, and social influences in your life. One of the most important factors in sexual healing is returning choice and consent to your sex life. Allowing yourself to discover what you like and enjoy sexually, and mending the self-blame and guilt that so often permeate desire, are both parts of the process of recovery.

> *I felt guilt for a long time about enjoying anal sex. I thought I was "acting out" the abuse because he raped me like that, and because it is unconventional, I think. Now I realize that I just like it. It feels good to me. I don't think I am acting out by liking kissing, and he did that, too.*—Marty

Somebody to Lean On: Self-Care and Support

You didn't get hurt alone, and you can't heal alone. Support is essential to any healing process. Isolation plays a key role in childhood sexual abuse. Most children never tell what is happening to them, and many who do tell are not believed or given adequate support. Adult survivors tend to continue to live in isolation. Coming out of isolation means coming into relationships. This, in and of itself, is a part of healing sexually.

Gaining support in your sexual healing breaks a double taboo. You will be talking not only about childhood sexual abuse but also about sex. While sex is overexposed in the media, we don't often sit down and tell each other the truth about our sex lives. Most people, survivors or not, have healing to do in the area of sexuality. The upside of this is that most people are relieved to talk about sex and sexual healing once someone else raises the topic. They, too, are glad to explore what is so often left unexamined.

Support includes both self-care and a community to be held by. Let's start with self-care.

Self-Care

Learning to care for yourself well is a lifelong journey. Your needs will change over time, and you will get better at it with practice. There are many different aspects of yourself to take care of: your body, your emotional and mental well-being, your financial life, your spiritual life, your family and relationships, your mission or meaning in life, your career, your sexuality, and your healing.

Here I am going to focus on the fundamentals of self-care. Attending to these fundamentals will give you a foundation to build upon during the challenging and exciting times of healing sexually.

EAT, DRINK, SLEEP, AND BE MERRY

Eating well can be a challenge for many survivors. Aim for two to three good meals a day, including plenty of fruits, vegetables, and protein. Drinking at least eight glasses of water a day will help your body flush out toxins that are released in the process of deep emotional work. Sleep regularly, seven to ten hours a night. And include pleasure in your life. What makes you smile or laugh? What brings that sense of warmth or comfort to your body? Perhaps you enjoy petting your cat, dancing, feeling the warmth of the sun, taking a luxurious hot bath… Do something pleasurable at least once per week. Notice your enjoyment.

LET YOUR BODY MOVE

Movement, including walking, biking, aerobic workouts, dancing, or running, can have a profound effect on your physical and emotional health. Movement oxygenates your body and increases your circulation. This helps in the process of healing and in relaxing. Whatever movement you choose, practice being "in" your body while you do it. Use this as a time to feel your breath and body sensations, rather than a time for checking out. This will assist you in being more embodied during all your activities, especially sex.

BREATHE

Breathing seems obvious, but it is not. Drop your breath lower in your body so that your diaphragm and chest move when you breathe. Notice when you are holding your breath, or breathing shallowly, and breathe deeply again.

TREAT YOURSELF WITH DIGNITY

How do you talk to yourself? Do you handle yourself with care and respect? Imagine how you would speak to a young child or a friend who is feeling afraid. You would not yell at her or tell her how stupid she is. Rather, you would be comforting, offering support and guidance. How you treat yourself internally is as important as what you do on the outside.

Give Yourself Lots of Acknowledgment

No one ever died from over-acknowledgment. Actively acknowledge yourself for your steps in healing. Notice all the risks you are taking, and give yourself support and kudos.

Make Time for Solitude

Solitude is also important to self-care. Make time for yourself weekly. You can use the time to write in a journal, sit quietly, do art work, meditate, or whatever else serves your process.

Incorporate Spirituality in Your Life

Many people also incorporate a spiritual practice or meditation into their lives. A spiritual practice can offer sustenance and a larger perspective to rest within. Meditation can be an excellent way to touch base with yourself, develop discipline, and learn to notice your own emotional processes. It is also a good way to learn to notice what is happening in your body, and to feel centered and at peace with yourself.

Deal with Addictions: Alcohol, Drugs, Food, Self-Deprivation

Many survivors have used food, alcohol, drugs, or self-deprivation as a means of coping with the sexual abuse. Many also use these substances to try to deal with sex. Some survivors cannot be sexual without getting high.

> *I couldn't have sex unless I was drunk or high. I would feel too out of control and triggered. The alcohol and drugs numbed that all out and gave me a kind of confidence. I had a lot of sex that I wouldn't really want to have today, though.—Lourdes*

I used drugs and alcohol to cushion myself from my feelings about the abuse. Alcohol helped me shut down. Alcohol helped me stay in sexually disappointing relationships for such a long time.—Max

If you have problems with substance abuse, get help. There are numerous recovery organizations to help you overcome addiction, including innovative programs like Recovery Systems Inc., a nutrition-based recovery program that attends to the effects of substance abuse and trauma on our physiology. Look in your local phone book for Twelve-Step programs like Alcoholics Anonymous and Overeaters Anonymous, as well as programs that employ numerous other approaches to recovery. See the Resources for more information.

Community Support

Community support includes all those who offer you love, care, information, guidance, and acceptance along the way. Community support may include friends, partners, co-workers, counselors and therapists, online buddies, self-help groups, supportive family members, and community groups. A varied support system offers more flexibility and availability—and a backup if your best friend is not around.

Support can be found by gaining referrals in your area from national survivors' organizations, speaking with friends and co-workers, checking newspapers and newsletters, visiting Internet chat rooms and joining newsgroups, or developing your own support group. Get creative in developing support.

I needed other women to talk to about my abuse and healing. I am a ritual abuse survivor, so this was especially terrifying, because of the stigma and because not a lot of people have very good information about it. After a lot of fear, I took a risk and started a ritual abuse peer support group. It is still scary, and it is exactly what I need.—Rose

Be clear with your support community about the focus of your healing. People can offer better support if they know what your journey and goals entail. Let your friends know that you are healing sexually now and what you may need from them. If you are uncertain at this time, you can inform them as you progress.

Sex-Positive Support

It has been challenging to find the community that can support me just as I am sexually. I found that my own exploration pushed a lot of people's buttons. I didn't want to be confined by my abuse or society's ideas of how I should be sexually. I think this was scary to people. People lacked information and education.—Rebecca

Because most of information available about sex in our society is negative and incomplete, it is likely that you are going to need to search out positive input about sex and your sexuality and preferences. Everyone can benefit from sex-positive information about human sexuality, the diversity of sexual expression, human sexual anatomy, and sexual development. It is likely that your support people, including most trained therapists, will also need sex-positive information.

The average physician receives less than twelve hours of sex education during her or his entire medical training. The average therapist, unless specializing in sexual "dysfunction," receives less than nine hours. By comparison, San Francisco Sex Information requires that potential hotline volunteers complete fifty-six hours of basic training in human sexuality. This is a thorough training and still barely begins to cover the information, experiences, and dynamics of human sexuality. For the most part, sex-positive information is not institutionalized but must be sought out.

A sex-positive, nonjudgmental attitude will be your most valuable asset in sexual healing. Sex for survivors can be laden with contradictions, guilt, and self-blame. Because sex was used against you as an instrument of harm rather than of healing, it is important to learn about the positive and self-affirming expressions of sex. You need support for exploring your desires at the same time that you are discovering the contradictions in your sexuality. It helps to have friends, counselors, and other supporters who can handle your wildest fantasies right along with the worst pain of your sexual abuse. It can be very damaging to get negative judgments about your sexual exploring, and it can be profoundly healing to find encouragement and acceptance as you become more empowered sexually.

Educating yourself and your supporters with sex-positive sex information can make all the difference.

Selecting a Therapist or Counselor

You are the boss of your own healing. You say how it goes. Although therapists are a help along the way, you get to decide what is best for you. You also get to ask for what you want and need from your support people. Your needs are likely to change as you change, so update yourself and your therapist as you proceed.

A good therapist for this type of healing work is one who has the capacity to be with you in the midst of the exciting and the ugly, someone who has done enough work on herself or himself to be able to travel in unknown territories with you. Experience in working with survivors is essential. Get a good sense of the therapist's attitudes about sex. Are her or his attitudes regarding sex strictly conventional, or can he or she support you in discovering your own sexuality? Watch out for narrow attitudes regarding homosexuality, S/M, pornography, and stereotypes about women's sexual expression. Is

Interviewing a Therapist

Here are some questions to ask a therapist you are considering as support for sexual healing:

- How many hours of training in human sexuality have you had?
- What do you consider the most important factors in sexual healing?
- Are you experienced in working with survivors of childhood sexual abuse? How have clients benefited from working with you?
- What do you see as the positive aspects of sex and sexual healing?
- What forms of sexuality do you consider dysfunctional?
- Do you hold religious beliefs regarding sex?
- Can you support my sexual healing in nonjudgmental way?
- What are your boundaries with clients?
- Are you willing to educate yourself further regarding sex and a sex-positive approach to healing for survivors?
- Do you have experience working with lesbian and bisexual women?
- Do you have experience working with transgendered clients?
- How do you feel about S/M, role-playing, porn, and rape fantasies?
- How do you feel about sex work?
- How do you feel about nonmonogamy and casual sex?
- Add your own questions.

your therapist familiar with the latest safer-sex guidelines? And is she willing to learn the things she may not know?

Most important, what kind of feel do you get from this person? Do your instincts say "Yeah!" or "Well…maybe…" or even "No"? Listen to these instincts.

While this may be obvious, I feel it is important to state that it is not appropriate for a therapist to have sex with his or her client. If you are invited into sexual contact with your therapist, end this therapeutic relationship and report the therapist to the police and the state licensing board.

Somatics: Including Your Body in Healing

My work is in *somatics*, an educational and transformational approach that assumes that the body, mind, and emotions are one interconnected biological system. You are not separate from your body; rather, your self is revealed in and through your body all the time. *Soma* is the Greek word for the living body, or thought, spirit, and body as one.

Many possibilities come from looking at the body this way. Instead of seeing the body as a carcass that we carry around, the body becomes an alive and intelligent presence. The body is not something to get away from but a source of wholeness to be returned to and embodied fully. In working with and through the body, trauma can be processed and completed, and pleasure, balance, and present time can be restored. In somatics the body becomes an inherent and essential part of the change and healing process.

In Western cultures we have inherited a worldview that sees our minds, emotions, and bodies as separate entities. This comes out of Western Cartesian philosophical views and Christian traditions that have considered thinking or mental functioning paramount. "Mind over matter," as the saying goes. Some religious beliefs even see the body as essentially sinful, something to be either ignored or controlled. These perspectives have begun to shift in the last fifty years in the West, with more exposure to indigenous and Eastern perspectives. Feminist theory and literature has critiqued this mind/body split and has encouraged a return to the knowledge and life of the body. Starting with Willhelm

Reich, Western philosophers and practitioners have also begun to reintegrate the body and mind.

Somatics recognizes an intelligence and life in the body that affects your thinking and your actions. If you change your body, or the "holding" or trauma in your body, then your thinking, your experience of the world, and often your identity will also shift.

Why a Somatic Approach to Healing Sexually After Childhood Sexual Abuse?

Childhood sexual abuse literally touches your body. To leave your body out of the healing process can leave out what is potentially your surest path to well-being. Many survivors of childhood sexual abuse are dissociated or "checked out" from their bodies. Your body was a dangerous place as a child. Leaving your body then, or dissociating, was an intelligent move. The memories or experiences of the trauma are often still present or "held" in your body today. Many survivors stay out of their bodies and senses long after the danger has passed to avoid revisiting those stored experiences.

Yet, your body is also *you*. It is the place in which you live and are alive. You connect and are in relationship with others from your body. You act in the world from your body. Your body is where the healing from trauma and abuse happens. Your body is also where you experience sensual and sexual pleasure. To experience all of these pleasures, however, you must be in your body, or "embodied."

Attending to the process of re-embodying is essential to sexual healing. I know it sounds strange, but building your tolerance for being in your body and experiencing physical pleasure is a central component of this healing. This is an intentional practice, especially in the beginning. After childhood sexual abuse, pleasure may be unfamiliar or uncomfortable to you.

> *I was surprised the first time I could stay present and embodied while my lover went down on me. It was like "Oh, this feels good. That's why people do this."—Carolyn*

Knowing your boundaries and having the ability to consent is also an embodied experience. If you are dissociated during sex, it is very difficult to know if you want to stop or go further or what sexual activities you want to consent to or invite.

Traditional psychoanalysis tends to focus on the mental processes, assuming the body will come along for the ride. This type of therapy has its place and can be useful for many, yet it can fall short of truly transforming the deep impact of sexual trauma. Most people have the experience of thinking one thing and doing another, even when they do not mean to. "Getting it" mentally does not necessarily translate into new ways of being or different actions. There can be an incoherence between your thinking and your body, because understanding something is different from embodying it.

> I know what I want sexually. I've read the books and have lots of ideas, but still when I get there my body freezes. It's like I can't keep track of what year it is and that I'm not a kid at home in my bed anymore.—Naomi

What I see in my work with survivors is that when they embody, when they return to life in their body and their sensations, a type of self-generated healing begins to happen. It is as if the body has not only a physical immune system but also an emotional and spiritual immune system or intelligence that orients towards health and balance. When you are dissociated from or ignore the body, this immune system does not function well. When the body is included, when the focus is on embodiment, the signs, signals, and functioning of this balancing system come into full swing. I have come to see the body, mind, and emotions as self-healing organisms when given the right conditions. Embodiment is one of these conditions.

I encourage including a body-based or somatic component to one's healing. I have found it one of the most efficient ways to process the abuse and release triggers. As you transform on the somatic level, the trauma is literally shifted and released, and you are able to live in present time, instead of being trapped in history, rage or depression. Somatics can help align your thinking, experience, and actions, bringing a sense of internal congruence.

There are a variety of somatic schools and modalities, including Strozzi Institute, Rubenfeld Synergy, and Somatic Experiencing. Further information can be found in the Resources at the end of this book. Other options for embodiment practices include dancing, martial arts, and body-focused meditation. Any practice that brings you regularly into your body and the sensations, feelings, and life of your body is useful.

Safer Sex

No chapter on safety in a sexual healing book would be complete without a discussion of safer sex. Safer sex is the practice of using barriers or limiting sexual activities to prevent the passage of bodily fluids from one person to another. Safer-sex techniques are used to prevent sexually transmitted diseases (STDs) including herpes, genital warts, HIV, chlamydia, and many others. The use of condoms is also effective in preventing pregnancy.

Use a Barrier

Most safer-sex barriers, such as condoms, latex gloves, dental dams, and female condoms, are made of latex, although there are others made from polyurethane and nitrile for folks who are allergic to latex. Lambskin condoms do not prevent HIV transmission, since the virus is small enough to pass through the membrane, and are not recommended for safer sex. For many, plastic food wrap is the barrier of choice for cunnilingus and analingus, as it is cheap, readily available, and easier to use than dental dams.

Don't Forget the Lubricant

Use a water-based lubricant with latex and other barriers—it will make the whole experience a lot more enjoyable. Water-based lubricant helps tremendously with the glide factor and increases sensitivity. Put some lubricant in the tip of the condom for the wearer and on the outside for more glide. Use lubricant on the receiver's side of the dental dam or plastic wrap during oral sex, and on the outside of the latex glove for a smoother touch.

Lubricants containing oil can weaken latex. Thus Crisco, Vaseline, and other oil-based lubricants are not recommended for use with condoms or any other latex product. Since I encourage the use of latex in preventing STDs, I recommend using only water-based lubricants.

Assess Your Risk

A lot of people speak of "risk factors" when discussing safer sex. To assess risk, you need to consider your own risk factors, those of your partners, and of the particular sexual acts you engage in. You can then choose what risks you feel are worth taking.

To assess your own risk, consider:

- the number of partners with whom you have had unprotected sex
- the number of partners *they* may have had sex with
- the risk level of your sexual activities
- your intravenous drug history
- your partners' intravenous drug history
- and if you currently have any STDs.

The more partners with whom you have had unprotected sex, the greater your risk level. If

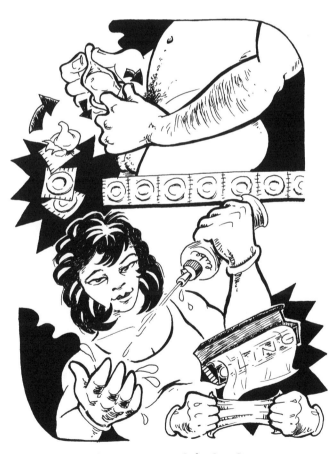

ILLUSTRATION 1. Safer-Sex Gear

you have used intravenous drugs, this also increases your risk. Of course, if you enjoy high risk sexual practices (for instance, unprotected anal intercourse), you should consider yourself at higher risk.

If you have any STDs or immune-deficiency disorders, you are at higher risk and may want err on the side of caution in your sexual practices to keep yourself well. Even if you are HIV-positive, you need to practice safer sex. First, having one strand of the HIV virus does not make you resistant to others. Second, exposure to other STDs can damage an already-compromised immune system.

When assessing your risk factors, remember that there is no guarantee that your partner is monogamous. Given the lack of permission to speak openly about having multiple sexual partners, many people will lie about it. Some people regularly have sex outside of a primary relationship without ever telling anyone. Your health is in *your* hands. While I am not asking you to be skeptical, I am encouraging you to be aware that you may not know all of your partner's sex history or current sexual practices. Have a conversation with your partner about safer sex and his or her sex and drug-use history. The best bet is to ask your partner to get tested for HIV and other STDs before you have sex together. Remember that HIV will probably not show up on tests for several months after exposure. A good practice is to get tested for HIV once every six months.

Play Safe

Some sexual practices are riskier than others. Semen and blood carry the highest concentration of the HIV virus, which can enter your bloodstream via small lacerations in the mouth, anus or vaginal tissues, or abrasions on the skin. Don't forget that HIV can be present in pre-cum and menstrual blood.

Other STDs, like herpes, can be transmitted through contact with open sores. However, just because you don't see an open sore on your partner's genitals does not mean you are free from risk. Some STDs, like HPV, are often symptom-free. And herpes can be transmitted just prior to an outbreak. (HPV, the virus that causes genital warts, has also been linked to cervical cancer.)

High risk sexual activities include unprotected cunnilingus during menstrua-tion (going down on a women during her period), unprotected anal intercourse and rimming (mouth-to-anus sex), and unprotected vagina/penis intercourse.

Vaginal fluids carry a lower concentration of HIV. So medium-risk behaviors include unprotected cunnilingus when a woman is not bleeding, unprotected fel-latio (giving head), and finger-fucking or fisting without a glove.

Low-risk behaviors include French kissing (wet kissing), hand jobs, protected penetration, and protected oral sex.

Sexual behaviors that are risk-free include tribadism (dry humping), fantasy, masturbation (only touching yourself), voyeurism and exhibitionism (watching or being watched). Phone sex and computer sex are also sexual activities free of the risk of STDs.

Use condoms on dildos, vibrators, and sex toys. Do not share your toys without changing the condom or cleaning them with an anti-bacterial cleanser. Remember that any toy you've used for anal play requires a fresh condom before you use it for vaginal play.

Check Yourself Out

Get a regular pelvic exam to care for your reproductive and sexual health. I know this is challenging for many survivors, but it is a *must do*, and a challenge worth taking on. Take a supportive friend with you. Advocate for yourself until you find a gynecologist who will listen to your needs. Your long-term health, including the prevention or early detection of cancer, depends upon you taking care of yourself in this way.

You can begin by getting tested for HIV and other STDs. You can find free, confidential testing in most cities though hospitals and STD clinics. Check your yellow pages and local newspapers. Ask your gynecologist to test you for STDs like herpes and chlamydia.

Make It Sexy

Many people are uncomfortable with using barriers at first. The best way to get comfortable with barriers is to go out and buy a bunch. Bring them home and play with them. Open the packages of condoms, female condoms, gloves, or dental dams and check them out. How do they feel, smell, taste? Become familiar with them—you'll lose your inhibitions. Practicing at home is often easier than practicing on your date! You can also eroticize latex and other safer-sex barriers. Soon the sound of your partner snapping on a latex glove will evoke memories of a very good time! Try including safer sex in your fantasies. How many ways can you find to make latex sexy?

Getting Started

Welcome to your continuing journey! The Sex Guide Exercises at the end of each chapter are designed to help you personalize and make use of the information in each chapter. They will help walk you through your process of sexual healing. I encourage you to share your process and discoveries with at least one other person. You can share your responses to the exercises or do them together.

> I think survivors who have done their healing have some of the best sex lives around. We have to look at, and deal with, heal, and redefine sex for ourselves. We do all this healing work that most people really need to do, survivors or not.—Stephanie

Sex Guide Exercises

Reflect on the following questions. Write about them in your journal and have a conversation about them with a support person.

1. Why heal sexually? What do you want to gain from it? How will your life be different and more satisfying? How will you know when you've gotten what you want?
2. What is safety to you? What is the difference between safety and comfort? What are examples of experiences in which you were safe yet uncomfortable?

3. Practice building an internal sense of safety. What sensations and feelings in your body give you a sense of safety, settledness, or resourcefulness? Where do you feel that now?

4. What support do you have now to assist you in your sexual healing?
    a. Self-care: journal writing, positive self-talk, ability to feel your emotions, eating well and exercising, somatic practices, spiritual practice.
    b. Community support: peer support group, therapist, friends you can talk to about sex and recovery.

5. What do you need to support your sexual healing? What actions can you take to build this network of support? Think big. Go beyond the bare minimum requirements for survival. Imagine having all the support you possibly could use. What would that be?

6. Take a look at your own attitudes and biases regarding sex. Make a list of what you think is healthy and not healthy regarding consensual sex. Discuss your list with a friend. Be sure to include issues of sexual orientation, what you consider appropriate sexual expression for women, fantasy, monogamy and nonmonogamy, abstinence, anal sex, religious beliefs, bondage, sado-masochism (S/M), cross-dressing, etc. This is an opportunity to explore your own beliefs about sex and sexual expression.

    Where do these ideas about sex come from? Where did you learn what you believe? Is there more for you to learn about anything on your list? Do you know anyone who practices any of the consensual activities that you listed as "not healthy"? This is an opportunity to explore and learn more about your own beliefs and values, those you want to keep and those you may want to change.

chapter two

Desire and Pleasure

Discovering Your Pleasure and Desire

Allowing yourself your own desire might not come naturally to you if you were sexually abused as a kid. Incest and childhood sexual abuse give you lots of practice in suffering, checking out, and enduring, and not a lot of experience of pleasure. You may have to learn to tolerate the feelings of pleasure and desire all over again.

Through sexual abuse, you learned to satisfy someone else's desires without your own boundaries, needs, or wants even entering the picture. You did not get the chance to experience the evolution of your own sexual desires, in your own time, based on your own needs. How, then, can you be familiar with your own desires now?

> *I am afraid to desire. I just take what comes and deal with that. That is what I do with sex, I realize, too. Whatever he wants…well, that's okay. It is too scary to think about what I want.*—Cindy

For some survivors, having *any* sexual desire is the first challenge. Your experiences may have convinced you that you are not allowed to have sexual pleasure or be happy and excited about your sex life. You may be convinced that liking sex as an adult means you must have liked it as a kid, too. If you liked it then, it wasn't really abuse, and this whole thing must be your fault, right?

I am just not turned on. I don't feel sexual desire.—Carla

Just so you know, this isn't true. Enjoying sexual pleasure does not make you bad and does not make the abuse your fault. Your sexual feelings are a testimony to your ability to hold onto yourself through extremely adverse conditions—and proof of your healing.

Components of your desire may scare you because they mimic the abuse you endured. You may find the dynamics of power and surrender to be a turn-on. Nothing is wrong with this. The difference between childhood sexual abuse and adult consensual sex is that in adult sex, *both* partners are matured sexually and have the ability to make choices for themselves. In consensual sex, you are not being coerced, manipulated, or misused. Both partners' needs, boundaries, and desires are considered.

> *I was orally raped as a girl. I really like oral sex today, but I feel guilty. Don't I just like this because I was abused this way?…I was abused almost every way you can have sex…so I guess that doesn't leave me many options.—Dede*

Those of us who have been sexually abused may mistake sexual energy for abuse itself. Part of your job in healing will be to learn to differentiate sex from abuse. Just like money, sexual energy can be used for beneficial or destructive ends.

A Depressed Libido

Many survivors experience depression as a symptom of sexual abuse. Some seek out antidepressants and other medication to help along the way. Most antidepressants decrease your sex drive. Many survivors taking antidepressants report little interest in sex, and an increased libido when they go off of the medication.

> *Anti-depressants did affect my libido. I wasn't as interested. I used it as a time, though, to learn about my sexuality, not being so intent on coming. I read sex information books, I touched and massaged my body, I became more sensual and really more sexual with myself. —Kathy*

If you are taking antidepressants or considering it, talk with your practitioner about their possible effect on your libido. You can try various types of anti-depressants to see which gives you the best results. For survivors who choose to stay on antidepressants long term, you can get a testosterone patch from your doctor, which tends to increase libido. Talk to your prescribing physician about your options and the side effects of both antidepressants and testosterone patches.

Luckily, finding and exploring your own desire is a learnable process, one that many people embrace as a lifelong commitment to themselves. First, come into your body, your feelings and sensations to find desire from the inside out. Then, educate yourself. What are all the different options for expressing my sexuality? What do people *do*, anyway?

Desire Is in Your Body

Your true desires reside in your body as feelings and sensations. Your sensations let you know that you are excited by someone, something, or an idea. When you shut down to avoid feelings of pain and betrayal, you also miss feelings of excitement, desire, and pleasure. Coming back into your body, reoccupying yourself from the inside out, is the most essential step in discovering your sexual desires. You *are* your body. Your thoughts take place in your body, along with your sensations, feelings, emotions, and even your spiritual longings and inspiration. Practice paying attention to physical feelings and sensations.

Let's say you are at work, sitting at your desk or standing behind the counter. Can you feel your legs? Your feet on the ground? What are the sensations you notice in your chest or stomach? Try this now. The next time you are feeling sexual pleasure or arousal, bring your attention into your body. Notice where in your body you feel sexual.

The Pelvic Rock

Lie on your back with your feet on the floor, knees bent. Place a mat or folded blanket underneath you so that you are comfortable. Let your body settle onto the floor and bring your attention into your body. Notice the sensations in your body. Drop your breath into your belly. Breathe deeply. Do this for at least three breaths before you start the rock.

Next, begin to slowly rock your pelvis forward and back. Bring your pubic bone toward your belly button, then rock it back toward the ground. Your lower back will press into the floor and then arch away from the floor. This looks like and might feel like a sexual motion. Slowly continue to rock your pelvis back and forth, focusing on staying in your body, feeling your sensations. Do this for at least three minutes.

You will probably have all kinds of responses to this. You might feel sexually aroused. Great! You might notice that you float out or start thinking about something else. Notice your thoughts, but don't let them draw your attention away from your feelings and the sensations in your body. Your emotional response to this exercise will give you information about what in you needs to heal. You may cry or get angry. Let that come, too.

Now match your breathing to the pelvic movement. Inhale as you arch your back and exhale as you bring your pelvis toward your belly button. You can try increasing the speed of the rocking. How does this change your response? Practice getting to a point where you feel slightly uncomfortable, and then stay with that feeling. This exercise will help you increase your tolerance for your own sexual energy and help you get in touch with your own desire. You will also free up your pelvis and genitals, allowing movement and sensation back into this part of you.

Genital Healing

Here is another exercise to help you come back into your body and your sexual desire. Again, lie comfortably on your back, with your knees up, feet on the floor. Settle onto the ground and into your body and sensations. Breathe into your belly, deepening your breath. Keep your attention on the feelings and sensations in your body.

Next, rub your hands together to bring some heat and energy into them. When you are ready, place one hand gently onto your genitals. Let the warmth of your hand radiate into your genitals and pelvis. You could imagine them thawing or relaxing, and more life returning to them. Imagine them healing. Keep breathing all the way down into your pelvis and genitals, and keep your attention in your body.

If you choose, you can place your other hand on your heart or over your lower abdomen just above your pubic bone.

Try this for five minutes per session.

Your Sexual Self-Education

Where did you learn about sex and desire? Who taught you about your body? What did your family, your abuser, your school or religious affiliations teach you about sex and about *your* sexuality in particular? Is this what you want to believe? Do you think the information you learned is correct? These questions provide a good beginning for your sexual self-education.

There are lots of ways now to increase your knowledge about sex and desire. For starters, the remainder of this book is filled with information about sex and various sexual styles. You can also learn about sex by talking to your friends. Ask them what they like, what they don't like, and why. Ask them what is easy for them about sex and what is difficult, and how their sex lives have changed over time. Most people are relieved to have an opportunity to talk honestly about sex and desire.

You can also read other people's accounts of sex. We are currently enjoying a boom in women's erotica. Annual series, such as *Best Women's Erotica*, edited by Violet Blue, *Best American Erotica*, edited by Susie Bright, and *Best Lesbian Erotica*, edited by Tristan Taormino, are great starting points for your research. You'll find stories featuring everything from suggestive sensuality to explicit S/M and bondage. Try reading about sex styles that attract you as well as those that differ from yours. Contact one of the sex toy retailers listed in the Resources for erotica suggestions. The Resources also lists many great sex manuals, such as *The Good Vibrations Guide to Sex* by Cathy Winks and Anne Semans. Here you can find positive and accurate sex information that treats sex as a normal part of being human. If you do not have access to erotica or sex manuals in your area, check out the mail-order companies listed in the Resources.

Watching erotic DVDs is another way to learn about sex and desire. You can find heterosexual, gay, and lesbian pornography. You can even find DVDs that match a special interest or fetish. And you can watch DVDs made by women like Candida Royalle, Nina Hartley, and Annie Sprinkle. Some of these look like traditional pornography and some have a very different aesthetic. There are also lesbians making pornography about lesbians—quite a leap from the traditional woman-on-woman sex scenes in mainstream pornography.

Some people try to make a distinction between pornography and erotica, but no one seems to be able to come up with definitions we can all agree on. I use the terms interchangeably.

Visit your friendly woman-run sex store to shop for erotic books and DVDs. The resource section of this book lists stores in New York, Boston, Toronto, Vancouver, Madison, Seattle, San Francisco, Austin, and other cities, along with "virtual shops" on the Web.

Virgins and Whores

Sexual desire and expression are amazingly diverse, varying vastly over time and from culture to culture. Ancient Chinese texts on sexuality noted twelve specific names for different depths of the vagina. Each was named for its unique sensation, and instructions were included on how to best touch that particular area. In the earliest of these texts, women were the teachers of sexual knowledge. In other tribal cultures, older women instructed young women in female ejaculation, orgasm, and different positions for sex in preparation for marriage and initiation into womanhood.

> **What Do You Think?**
>
> People have strong opinions about pornography. Here's mine: I do not find anything "wrong" with sex on film. Porn can be hot, interesting, and erotic. The complications come when we look at the context in which porn is made. We still live in a society in which women earn far less than men for the same work. Children who report sexual abuse are not believed, rape victims are put on trial, and sexually powerful women are suspect.
>
> The pornography industry for the most part is run by and profits men. There are abuses perpetrated against women in the pornography industry, as in many others. Yet many talented women work in the sex industry by choice as directors, producers, and actresses. The key issues, for me, are consent and economic independence. My wish for women in the sex industry is that they profit from their work—personally and financially—and fully enjoy sexual self-determination.
>
> What do you think?

In the West, views on sex and desire have changed over time as well. In the early twentieth century, vibrators were sold to physicians as medical devices that were used on women to cure "hysteria." Basically, women were going to the doctor for an orgasm. Vibrators later became novelty items, and now very few people tell the sales clerk just what they are going to use that new back massager for!

Most of us are familiar with the model of women's sexuality that permits us to be either virgins or whores. As women, we are not supposed to like sex, much less be fully expressed sexually on our own terms. (Quite a radical thought, huh?) A sexually expressed woman is considered a whore. Yet while we are not supposed to relish our own pleasures, we are supposed to be compelling sexual creatures, satisfying our partners. We are constantly acknowledged or disregarded in relation to our sexual desirability. This is quite a contradictory and confusing message.

In fact, the word *virgin* in its root definition means "she who is not owned by another." Being virginal in its authentic definition has nothing to do with having had sex or not. A virgin is a woman who is self-possessed. May we all develop virginal sex lives.

> *First I had to wade through what my perpetrators told me about sex. Then I had to sort through the church and my neighborhood, what they think. It came off like layers, and I saw more and more of me. The piece I am working with now is my own "off-limits" territory around sexuality. There are these places I want to explore but am afraid to let myself. It keeps coming back to me being like them [the perpetrators] if I really like sex.—Sheila*

What's even crazier is that the sexual norms we inherit bear little resemblance to what people actually *do*. I think it would be great if everyone told the truth—for one moment—about their *actual* sexual practices and relationships, affairs and arrangements, fantasies and desires. The diversity would amaze us all.

We are still taught that heterosexuality is the norm and that only a few people practice same-sex eroticism. Yet in 1990, The Kinsey Institute reported that 35 to 50 percent of men and about 55 percent of women had same-sex erotic experiences.

While we are *slowly* changing our expectations of lifelong, monogamous, heterosexual marriage as the norm, the fact is this has not been the practice of most people for centuries. Today, most people practice serial monogamy and non-monogamy. We can look at divorce rates and media coverage of extramarital affairs for evidence of this. Look at your own circle of friends and colleagues to get the picture. Some people practice consensual nonmonogamy, also called *polyamory*, an arrangement that is chosen by the primary partners in a sexual relationship. Sadly, most people still practice the nonconsensual kind.

The Complexity of Desire

Desire is not a tidy little package that stays consistent over time. Desire in fact is multifaceted and full of contradictions.

This can be particularly true for survivors of childhood sexual abuse. I find that many survivors try to rid themselves of these contradictions in an attempt to make their desires simpler, more "normal." I am not sure that anyone's sexuality is "normal" in the sense of matching cultural agendas. Human sexuality is more complex than the stereotypes imply.

Healthy sexuality embraces contradiction. This means that two or more seemingly opposite emotions or desires can be held at the same time. You may feel intense desire and shame at the same time. Sex and desire for you may hold both guilt and ease. You may want to be loved tenderly, to touch softly and be held, while another part of you wants to bite, whip, or tie someone up.

> It is weird with pornography...sometimes it really turns me on and other times I find it rather repulsive. I feel this way about some of the more intense and rough sex I have. I love it in the mix and feel guilty afterward sometimes. I try not to judge it anymore or try to find the "right" answer. I try to give myself room for all of it.—Melanie

Owning Your Desire

Sex is one of those aspects of human experience that everyone has an opinion about. Lots of people and institutions—such as your family, church or synagogue, the media, and even your women's rugby team—will be happy to tell you what your desires are or should be. What it comes down to is this: Will you decide for yourself or have someone else do it for you? You may take some heat if your desire

Sexual Diversity

Bisexual: Having sexual desire, interest, and/or activity with people of both sexes.

Celibate: Choosing to not engage sexually with another and/or with oneself.

Gay: Having sexual desire, interest, and/or activity with people of one's own sex; often refers specifically to men.

Heterosexual: Having sexual desire, interest, and/or activity with people of the opposite sex.

Lesbian: For women, having sexual desire, interest, and/or activity with other women.

Marriage: A legal and/or social contract declaring an emotional and financial commitment to a relationship. In most of the world, only heterosexuals are allowed to be married legally.

Monogamous: Choosing to be sexual with only one other person.

Nonmonogamous: Choosing to be sexual with more than one other person.

Pansexual: Having sexual desires, interests, and behavior with all genders, sexual orientations and persuasions. Many people embrace this term in an attempt to broaden the categories of gay and straight, man and woman, S/M and vanilla.

Polyamorous: *Poly* means many and *amor* love. Choosing to have sexual relations with more than one person. Some people prefer this term to nonmonogamous.

S/M: Sadomasochism is a sexual practice which can include power play, intense sensation, pain, bondage, and role playing.

Serial monogamy: Engaging in a series of monogamous sexual relations, one after the other.

Tantra: A sexual practice which views sex as a sacred path of spiritual transcendence.

Transgendered: An umbrella term, including transsexuals and transvestites, as well as others who identify as being differently-gendered. A transgendered person may identify as gay, heterosexual, lesbian, or pansexual.

Transsexual: A person who identifies with and lives as a gender other than that assigned at birth. Transsexuals usually engage in some form of altering the physical body, such as hormone therapy or gender reassignment surgery. Female-to-male transsexuals (FTMs) identify as men, and male-to-female transsexuals (MTFs) identify as women. A transsexual may identify as gay, heterosexual, lesbian, or pansexual.

Transvestite: A person who cross-dresses.

Vanilla: A term used by S/M practitioners to describe non-S/M sex.

falls outside of the heterosexual, monogamous, married, missionary-position style for your sexual expression. Well, most people's desires fall outside of this narrow frame. No wonder we so rarely speak up about our sexual desires! Even if married, missionary-position sex is your favorite—which is fine—you may have other desires that don't fit this expression.

Following are some examples of what some women find desirable.

Sexual Activities

admiring asses
anal sex
being penetrated deeply
being tied up
biting my lover's breasts
caressing a lover to orgasm
cross-dressing
cyber sex
double penetration
dressing slutty
dripping hot wax on someone's skin
erotic dancing
exhibitionism
eye contact
fantasizing about making love
fisting
flirting
foot worship
French kissing
fucking
genderplay
getting a piercing or tattoo
getting head
giving head
golden showers

group sex
hair pulling
hand jobs
having my breasts stroked
having my ear and neck licked
having sex while blindfolded
holding hands
hugging
intercourse
kissing
kissing my partner's nipples
kneeling
looking at my lover's body
massage
masturbating with a vibrator
modeling for erotic photos
orgasm
outdoor sex
phone sex
playing with butt plugs, alone or with a partner
playing with feathers
playing with ice cubes
playing with nipple clamps
playing with riding crops
playing with Saran wrap

putting on a condom
reading erotic fiction
reading sex manuals
rimming
role-playing
shaving
spanking
talking about sex with friends
talking about sex with potential sex partners
tickling
tying up my lover
using dildos and harnesses
using sensual oils
voyeurism
watching erotic DVDs
wearing a man's suit and tie
wearing corsets and sexy lingerie
wearing leather
wearing rubber/latex clothing
whipping
wrestling
writing in a journal about sex

People used to think that the world was flat. That is how I was about sex. I thought sex was a sin and bad. When you stand in the plains, the world does look flat; you have to look from a bigger perspective to see that the world is round.—Rona

I sometimes feel that my sexual desires are bad, grotesque, abnormal. This is connected to what I think a woman should be—my desires seem "unladylike." —Louisa

Like other things we take for granted, our views on sex are influenced by social and historical forces, along with cultural heritage and religious beliefs. There is no "right" way of having consensual sex; rather, there are options you may or may not choose. Which options help to heal you? Which empower and support you? Owning your desire means that you take responsibility for discovering what fits for *you* sexually. You get to be the one who names the unique sexual expression that is yours. Grant your*self* permission.

It was so amazing when I realized that I could really set up my sex life however I wanted to…that I could run my sex life by my own rules. I had always felt too guilty to like sex. What I really wanted was to date a number of people at once, and I wanted to explore sexually. I did not know anything about me and what I liked and wanted. I wanted to find out, so I started. Nonmonogamy has been amazingly freeing for me. Oh, and I practice safe sex, too.—Rebecca

Sex Guide Exercises

Write about the following. Then, have a conversation with a friend or therapist about what you wrote.

1. Take a sexual self-inventory. What have you experienced sexually up to now? What did you like? What did you not like? What do you know about your sexuality? What would you like to learn?

2. Take a piece of paper and make three columns, titled "yes," "maybe" and "no." In the "yes" column, list all the sexual activities that you enjoy or think you would enjoy. In the "maybe" column, list all the sexual activities that you enjoy under certain circumstances or that you might be willing to try. In the "no" column, list all the sexual activities that you do not enjoy and do not want to explore. Include both masturbation and partner sex. Now, look at your lists. Which column most closely resembles your current sex life?

3. Imagine an activity that is physically pleasurable to you, enlivening to your senses. It could be walking on warm sand, feeling the breeze against your face, touching your partner, having oral sex. Imagine yourself in that scene now. What kinds of sensations are you feeling while you experience this specific pleasure? Where in your body do you feel them? How much pleasure or desire can you take in?

4. What sexual activity or fantasy would you like to try out? Be explicit. What's stopping you?

chapter three

Dissociation

What do you, mean be in my body for sex? I spend my energy trying not to be there during sex.—Hannah

What I am really best at sexually is checking out. I can do it through fantasy, thinking about fixing the car, or wondering what school my kids should go to— and I don't even have kids yet...—Kathy

Checking Out

Dissociation is "checking out." It is crawling out of your skin to get away when there is no other way to get away. Dissociation is a normal and healthy response to trauma. It is a creative and self-preserving attempt to manage the experience of being abused. As a child, you tried to distance yourself mentally, emotionally, and spiritually from the pain, manipulation, and betrayal of sexual abuse. Dissociation is a survival tool, and a good one at that. You would not have survived as intact as you are had you not dissociated.

I have come to think of dissociation as a kind of emotional immune system response. When a virus invades your body, your immune system acts automatically to preserve your health. You do not have to send out any kind of alert or instructions. Dissociation also happens without us thinking about it or having control over it.

People experiencing very different types of traumas report the same experience of dissociation. Survivors of domestic violence and rape, war veterans, political prisoners, and torture survivors all use dissociation as a survival tool. If the trauma or betrayal is too much for the psyche to process at that time, some level of distancing from the event takes place.

Dissociation over Time

The funny thing about dissociation is that it is a temporary survival technique. Although you get away from the immediate pain and fear, the trauma does not get processed or healed by dissociating. It remains with you, to be attended to at a safer time. Dissociation is designed to get you through and out of the traumatic event. The healing of the trauma comes later.

The emotional responses to sexual abuse remain in your body, awaiting your attention. During recovery you have the chance to reintegrate, to feel and come to peace with these bodily held traumatic experiences. You may experience a kind of thawing out as you return to yourself, melting back into your own body and reoccupying your own skin.

A tricky thing about dissociation is that it can continue long after the danger is over and its usefulness has passed. Dissociation becomes so practiced that you can find yourself leaving your body even when you are not in danger.

> The ordinary response to atrocities is to banish them from consciousness. Certain violations of the social compact are too terrible to utter aloud: this is the meaning of the word *unspeakable*.
>
> The psychological distress symptoms of traumatized people simultaneously call attention to the existence of an unspeakable secret and deflect attention from it. This is most apparent in the way traumatized people alternate between feeling numb and reliving the event.
>
> —Judith Lewis Herman, M.D., *Trauma and Recovery: The Aftermath of Violence—From Domestic Abuse to Political Terror*

I have found so many "parts" of me that have no idea that the abuse has ended. They are on continuous red alert, awaiting the next attack.—Shandell

Many survivors come to believe that being dissociated—or out of your body—is the safest and sometimes the *only* safe way to live. Even if you *know* you are safe, dissociation may still be your automatic response to closeness, intensity, fear, or sexuality. Dissociating comes to be what feels natural.

I still sometimes find myself floating outside of my body as if I am walking behind myself. This happens particularly when I am scared or startled. It's like it is automatic, the first place I know to go to feel safe.—Henrietta

Dissociation: How It Works

Dissociation happens in lots of ways that are actually fairly predictable. Some survivors report floating out of their bodies and watching the abuse from the other side of the room. Others talk about going deep inside to a very small place, where no one could find them, touch them, or get them.

My brother abused my sisters and me. I remember several times I had out-of-body experiences. I felt as if I were sitting on the window sill, watching. That's also what I felt like when I started having sex. I just wasn't there.—Marie

My baby-sitter abused me when I was in first and second grade. He said it was a game and that I'd like it. He'd make me change into my nightgown and do a headstand against the wall. Then he'd stick his fingers in my vagina. I bought his story. I abandoned myself by not trusting my own instricts and feelings about what was happening.—Louisa

Still others tell about focusing on a very small speck on the ceiling or singing or talking themselves into another world.

I would hear my dad walking across my bedroom. I would face the wall pretending I was asleep, holding my eyes closed tight. No one taught me how to do this, but spontaneously in my mind I would start chanting, "This isn't happening, this isn't happening, this isn't my dad, this isn't my dad." Over and over again I would do this. This would help me leave, go into some kind of altered state.—Carla

My father often molested me after dinner when I was in my room doing school-work. Reading and schoolwork became my main means of escape. I would just focus on the reading or the math problem until he finished and go back to my schoolwork. I became so adept at this that one time I hardly set down the book.—Akaya

We do things with our bodies to dissociate. Pretend you are scared or star-tled—what happens? Most likely you tense your muscles and hold your breath. Dissociation usually involves shallow breathing or holding your breath. Holding your breath sends your body into a form of shock. Tensing and holding your mus-cles constricts the flow of blood and can numb sensations. When you are under attack or afraid, adrenaline courses through your body. This also helps to numb sensation and sends your body into a fight, flight, or freeze response.

I would freeze whenever my uncle picked me up. My body would get tense all the way down to the bone. It was like he touched me and I quit breathing.—Liz

Some survivors dissociated from the feelings of the abuse but visually remem-ber exactly what happened. Many of these survivors believe that the abuse was "no big deal." By dissociating from their feelings during the abuse, they tried to minimize its emotional impact.

I always remembered what my mom would do to me and my brother. I just shrugged my shoulders like, "Whatever…she was just weird." What I didn't get is that there was actually a reason behind me feeling like I was tainted or some-thing was wrong with me. There was a reason I did so many drugs and had sex with so many people.—Carolyn

Dissociation can be as subtle as "spacing out" for a brief time or as extreme as blocking the memory of the abuse entirely. This is called traumatic amnesia. You may have no recollection of the abuse whatsoever or only a vague sense that something happened. Or, you may know that you are terrified of a certain person or place—but have no idea why.

As the dissociation thaws, memories can return in many ways. You may experience "body memories," actually experiencing the pressures, sensations, and terror of the abuse, yet having no visual or narrative recollection of the events. You may remember disjointed pieces of information—places, people, or specific details. Some survivors have a full-video replay, remembering sights, sounds, feelings, and even smells. The specific type of recollection matters less than the healing that comes from it. Re-embodying and thawing from dissociation are vital to healing your sexuality. The numbers and types of memories are less significant.

Every survivor I have worked with minimizes the abuse in some way. "It was worse for someone else," "I should be over it," "What's the big deal? He just made me suck him off," are comments I hear over and over again. Minimizing sexual abuse is another means of dissociating or distancing yourself from the pain. To really acknowledge the impact of childhood sexual abuse, to really face how it has affected your life, means feeling the pain, anger, loss, and betrayal. The good news is that this heals you—*and* it gets you in touch with the enormous resources, resilience, and courage that got you through.

Dissociation and You

How can you tell when you are dissociated *now?* The ways that you dissociated in the past to survive the abuse are most likely the ways that you continue to dissociate today. It's as if your nervous system learned a certain route and uses it again and again to bring you to safety. This can be frustrating when you consciously know that you are safe and that the person you are having sex with is not your perpetrator, and *still* you respond by dissociating. Your body is responding from habit.

The good news about this automatic dissociation is that you can learn to notice how it works and then work with it. As you learn what happens for you when you dissociate, you can learn how to find your way back.

To start, consider what it's like when you check out. Where do you go? What are you thinking? What do you say to yourself? How does the world look to you when you are dissociated?

Following are examples from survivors:

When I am dissociated, the vividness of things fades. The colors are less bright and everything feels distant or separate from me.

Instead of telling the truth, I try to make everything look okay. It feels like I am the only one who knows what is going on, and I'm faking out my lover. This is how I can tell that something must have scared me and I am going into survival mode.

I am easily distracted, thinking of everything other than the sex I am having, like figuring out who's going to baby-sit the kids next week, and what I should do about a problem at work. I start to think a lot.

I can't really feel my body anymore. I feel like I am floaty. I can't find me. Sometimes I look down at my arm and wonder if that is really mine.

I hold my breath and just go blank. I can't think or feel.

Your Body and Dissociation

Now look for the body process that goes along with dissociation for you. What is happening in your body when you dissociate? Watching your breath is usually a good place to start. Is your breath shallow? Are you holding your breath?

What about the rest of your body? Can you feel your arms and legs? Do you feel any sensation in your back? Are you tensing the muscles in your shoulders, pelvis, or genitals? Does your lower body disappear? Scan through the rest of your body. Which places in your body are blank or frozen? Which areas do you not want to inhabit?

I hold my breath and tense up around my chest. Then, internally, it's like I am running around looking for a safe place to hide. My adrenaline starts pumping.
—Jeanie

*I make the muscles around my pelvis and genitals really tight when I am afraid and start to space out. This usually goes along with holding my breath.
—Jennifer*

You may find that you have little or no sensation in a particular part of your body. It may feel blank, numb, or void. This is an area to pay attention to. It may hold old tension and trauma from the abuse.

I have this idea that I don't have genitals. There is a brain part and a body part, and the body part, particularly my genitals, is detatched.—Terri

I can hardly focus on my lower back and ass. I can stay there for a millisecond, and then I realize I've checked out again.—Rona

The Trigger

What caused you to dissociate? Can you trace your experience back to the moment where you started dissociating? What did you want to get away from? These questions may seem unanswerable at first. You may think, "I don't know, it just happens." You can learn to notice, however.

I was masturbating and realized I was checking out. I stopped and tried to see when I started to go away. I realized that as soon as I began to feel sexy and move my hips, I felt a wave of shame and then wanted to get away.—Stephanie

Usually, dissociation is a move away from some overwhelming or uncomfortable sensation or emotion. Your body registers a feeling you perceive to be dangerous or threatening and helps you remove yourself to safety. Now that you are an adult and engaged in a process of healing, you are no longer in danger, however much you may feel afraid. Feeling these emotions and moving toward these sensations is your path to healing and having your life and sexuality back.

By learning what happens in your body when you dissociate, you can come to know the intricacies of how and when you check out. This then gives you options for how to check in again. Eventually you can learn how to notice dissociation as it is happening and not check out at all. You can develop a habit of bringing *you* back to yourself over and over again. You will find that you return more quickly and easily with practice.

The Road Back: Healing Dissociation

While dissociation helps you survive sexual abuse, coming back into yourself allows you to experience the full spectrum of being alive. Returning to your body lets you be there for sex. If you are not present, how can you feel pleasure, connect with your partner, or even know what you want?

> *For a long time life felt safer if I was in my head. I didn't want to feel my body or my feelings because it was too scary and out of control. Too much of the abuse would come up. I fell for this guy, though, and it was so hard to feel him deeply. I couldn't feel much sexually and it was hard to stay there for it. I knew I loved him, and I couldn't stand not being able to feel more. Finally it became worth it to me to learn how to be here.—Jeanette*

Tracking

As you begin to notice the various ways you dissociate and what that state is like for you, you'll probably find a pattern or rhythm to it. You may find a consistent response in your body that lets you know you are on your way out. You may also find that when you dissociate, you say things to yourself, like "nothing matters anyway" or "I am worthless." These patterns become recognizable and thus easier to notice and work with.

Review what you have discovered about your own dissociation. What are the sensations in your body that go along with checking out? Notice again the places in your body you are dissociated from, areas that are blank, numb, or frozen. What do you tell yourself when you go away? What sends you out? Begin to track your own route of dissociating.

Here are some examples:

First I hold my breath. I lose track of most of my body and can only feel my head and shoulders. My thinking gets really fast. It is like I start to run around inside looking for a safe place to be. The world outside of me disappears and I get very internal.

I get tense all over, but especially in my shoulders and through my pelvis. My breathing is shallow, and I start to try to be really good. I kind of lose myself and pay attention to reading other people…What do they want from me? How should I act? I lose the internal sense of myself and get very other-focused.

My body will feel like it is something attached to me or not mine at all. I look down at myself and do not relate. I feel hazy or like my head is swimming. It is kind of scary. I notice that what triggers me is usually some emotion that gets too intense. It can be anger or pleasure.

My arms and neck get very tense. My jaws, too. I also get angry and annoyed at everything. I just want to push things and people away. I want it all to get away from me. It is like I want to get rid of all internal and external stimulation…have everything stop.

Knowing your own dissociative states lets you recognize where you are. From there, you can learn to come back. A wonderful friend of mine once said, "To heal, you first have to become intimate with what is." Knowing what you are like when you check out is doing just this.

Returning

Noticing that you are checking out is half the battle. Watch for your own signals, particularly those sensations that let you know you are going away. Once you notice, drop your breath low in your body, down into your belly. Breathe. Reassure yourself. Tell yourself everything is going to be all right. Invite yourself back.

Get up and move your body. Increase your blood flow and heart rate by swinging your arms or shaking your legs. Bring your focus back into your body. If you can't feel a particular area of your body, rub yourself there. Bring the feeling back into you. Notice your surroundings. What color are the walls? Who is in the room with you?

Then bring your focus to your emotions. What are you feeling? Say this out loud: "I am scared" or "I am sad." Do you need to tell someone what's going on? Do you need support? Believe it or not, you will survive your fear, anger, pleasure, and grief.

Emotions show up as sensations in the body. When you feel shame, what physical sensations go along with that? What about guilt? Or pleasure? Or love? What is it like to feel the emotion instead of making it go away? To embody, you must build your tolerance for more intense sensations. To have an embodied sex life, you must learn to face the feelings you needed to turn away from in the past.

Last, watch what you are thinking. Are the messages you are telling yourself soothing or empowering? Or self-denigrating? Often we are hard on ourselves as a way of avoiding feelings of anger, hurt, or fear. It may seem easier to be cruel to yourself than to face what others did to you. This internal cruelty helps to keep you dissociated. If you find you are speaking harshly to yourself, try telling yourself something neutral ("Breathe. It's okay. I am going to be okay.") or even positive if you can get there ("I'm worth it. I can do this.")

Embodiment Practices

Most important, consciously practice being embodied. Dedicate time to it. Working with dissociation is working with re-embodiment. You can increase your tolerance for the rushes of shame, pleasure, anger, and love that once sent you into dissociation. This is a process of building your capacity to be present for your sensations and emotions.

FIVE MINUTES:
Practice noticing the sensations in your body, including your legs, arms, and genitals, for five minutes each morning. What do you notice? Which feelings and sensations are easier for you to tolerate and which are more difficult? Notice where you want to turn toward a sensation and where you want the sensation to go away. Stay as long as you can with the ones you want to get rid of.

BELLY BREATHE:

Notice when you hold your breath or breathe very shallowly. Stop and breathe deeply and regularly again. Breathe down into your belly so that your stomach and chest move. You may notice yourself not breathing fifty times a day. That's okay; in fact, it is great that you notice. This is how you will retrain your automatic responses.

MOVE YOURSELF:

Physical activities such as walking, biking, and swimming are helpful in the practice of being embodied. This is physical activity not for exercise, but rather as a practice of getting to know your body more intimately. As you move, bring your attention to your sensations and senses. How do your arms feel? Your legs? How about inside your chest and stomach? Is it warm or hot or cool? Do you notice a twitch? Do you feel relaxed?

BODYWORK:

I encourage anyone healing from sexual abuse to engage in therapeutic bodywork. This is not massage to work your muscles, but bodywork that serves to open the frozen or armored places in your body. Therapeutic bodywork attends to the emotions as well as the body, allowing you to come back into your body and live in it gladly. See the Resources for information on a variety of therapeutic bodywork styles.

EMBODIMENT PRACTICES:

Centering practices, such as martial arts, yoga, dance, and some forms of meditation, can help you build your capacity to be in your body. Again, this is not about pushing yourself physically, but rather about developing a place of centeredness in your body and an awareness of your body. You can learn that being relaxed and being empowered can happen at the same time. Being embodied and being safe can exist simultaneously.

This might sound strange, but I've been learning that if I stick around to feel both my body and my heart, I'm not going to die. I thought that I would.—Roslyn

Coming back to our bodies can be terrifying, mostly because we have come to associate being in our bodies with danger, pain, terror, and betrayal. Who would want to be there? In the past, dissociating was an excellent survival strategy to get away from the abuse. The difference now, however, is that the abuse is over, and along with pain, anger, and loss, we get to feel pleasure, delight, ease, and connection.

I can notice when I start to hold my breath or feel a rush that once would have been too much. I relax in the moment now, breathe, feel the sensations, remind myself that it is okay to feel. I am here with me. Then I am back. I do this during sex!—Maggie

Talk About It

Talk with others survivors about what it is like when they dissociate. It can be very useful to compare notes. They may recognize something in their pattern of dissociating that you haven't noticed in yours.

My girlfriend started noticing me spacing out during sex before I would. She'd ask, "Where are you now?" I was surprised. I didn't realize I had gone any-where.—Janie

Often, your intimate partner will notice that you are dissociating before you do. If your partner is not aware of your dissociation, it's important that he or she learn to recognize the signs that you are checking out. Try talking to your part-ner about dissociation now; it's easier to talk about it when you are not in the throes of it, making it easir to bring up when you are triggered.

My husband and I had to find a balance between him checking in with me and him interrupting the flow of sex. Sometimes I had to tell him to shut up and quit asking me if I was present. I think half of my annoyance, though, was him bringing me back to the present, which was a much scarier place to have sex from.—Sally

Sex Guide Exercises

1. Explore what being dissociated or "checked out" is like for you. What happens in your body when you dissociate? What do you say to yourself internally?

2. How can you recognize this state for yourself? How could a partner or friend help you recognize it? What would they sense or see in you when you dissociate?

3. What do you have to gain by living an embodied life? What do you have to gain by having an embodied sex life?

4. List three ways you can begin to re-enter your body, or re-associate. What embodiment practices are you willing to take on regularly?

chapter four

Self-Denial

Self-denial is not behaving in accordance with your needs and desires. Self-denial is brushing your wants under the rug over and over again, not putting in your two cents' worth, not asking the world to include and adjust to you, too. Self-denial is not letting you be *you*.

> *I know what I want sexually, but I am too afraid to ask or say. I feel like I am imposing. Like I am not supposed to have needs or desires.*—Hannah

Being sexually abused as a kid teaches you that your needs and desires are unimportant and that your body and sexuality exist for someone else's use. Abuse tells you that your boundaries are wrong—or at least ineffectual. After childhood sexual abuse, many survivors are left feeling little or no permission to have desires, needs, or boundaries, or to take up space.

> *I don't assume I deserve anything, really. I adjust to the room I'm in and the people I am with. I think I am always watching for how I am supposed to act so that I won't be hurt again.*—Mimi

Sexual abuse tells you that you are not supposed to be delighted and fulfilled. You may feel guilty when you feel pleasure, thinking that you must be bad or that your pleasure denies someone else theirs. Shame, self-blame, and suffering become familiar, and pleasure and fulfillment become suspect.

As a survivor, you may find that you deny or minimize your sexuality alto- gether. Or you may find that sex is all you think you are good for. Respectively, these are called sexual aversion and sexual compulsion.

All I want to do is get sex away from me. I do not want to have sex or to be sexual. I think that the world would be a better place if sex did not exist. I could feel safe then.—Amy

Sex is what I know best. It is the way I know how to interact; sometimes it seems like the only way I know. When I want comfort, I have sex. When I am lonely, I have sex. Sometimes when I am hungry, I have sex to try to deal with it. When I just want to get to know someone as a friend, I find myself in bed with them. Sex has become my interface with the world.—Maggie

Many therapeutic models still pathologize sexual aversion and compulsion as types of "dysfunction." This framework says that something is "wrong" with you, instead of as seeing your sexual strategies as creative means of survival. Whether you've leaned toward sexual avoidance or sexual compulsion, you've done what- ever you needed to do to survive. These choices were intelligent at the time. They were survival-smart. Congratulate yourself.

Survival Is a Powerful Act

Survivors often have a lot of self-judgment about their own sexuality. You may be angry at yourself for avoiding sex for so many years or pissed about how many times you have had sex when you needed something else instead. It can be hard to accept our own survival strategies. Recovery asks us to hold the contradiction of having acted in ways that have hurt us while we were attempting to achieve some kind of self-preservation.

Whatever you did to survive sexual abuse, to be able to go on, is powerful. If avoiding sex helped you to stay safe, that's okay. If you had sex when and with people you did not want, that's okay. Nurture both self-compassion for your past choices and responsibility for taking care of yourself now.

I knew that I didn't want to have sex with all the men I was having sex with, but I didn't know how to stop. I would tell myself, "Not this time, this time I'm not going to have sex with him," and would find myself in bed with him. I was so hard on myself for doing this. It felt like I was permanently flawed. —Melanie

I felt ashamed after a while that I wasn't interested in sex at all. It seemed the entire world revolved around this thing I couldn't relate to. I sometimes felt superior and at the same time damaged—like what is wrong with me?—Laurie

Sexual Aversion: Who Needs Sex, Anyway?

After my grandfather started molesting me I became hypersensitive to anything sexual. I couldn't make him stop, but I sure as hell was not going to let anyone else touch me. I became rigid and afraid of anything sexual.—Marianne

Many survivors attempt to manage the intensity of emotion, triggers, and memories that can come up during sex by avoiding sex altogether.

It took me a lot of healing to get down into what drove my disinterest in sex. I knew it was related to the incest, but I only got it in my head, which wasn't allowing me to change much. Finally, I connected to the feelings of it all. Being sexual and opening sexually revealed to me the devastating pain and grief of the abuse. Keeping sex out of my life for the most part was helping me avoid all of those feelings. To be sexual I needed to also feel the impact of the abuse and heal there.—Danielle

By avoiding sex, you may also think you can avoid destructive beliefs about yourself that you learned from the abuse. If you were taught that you are only good for sex, avoiding sex could seem to prove that this is not true. If you were taught that the abuse was all your fault, avoiding your sexuality could seem to help you avoid the deep shame and guilt that comes with that.

My guilt about the sexual abuse runs so deep. If I have a good time sexually, I feel like I am betraying someone—or it proves that I wanted the abuse all along. It is easier not to have sex.—Rona

You may be afraid that if you express your sexual energy it will be too big or overwhelming and harm you or someone else. You may associate sex and being turned on with perpetration. You may associate your own sexual expression with being abusive.

There is a certain amount of intensity in my sexuality. I get afraid that the intensity will verge on rage. I have never hurt someone else sexually, but I try to keep myself under lock and key. Am I trustworthy, or will I be just like them [the perpetrators]?—Stephanie

You may be sexual but not fully expressing the sexual energy that is yours. This too becomes a type of sexual aversion, a denial of your sexuality.

I used to let my relationships define my sexuality. If my lover wasn't into penetration, then it didn't happen much. If my lover recoiled at the thought of vibrators and dildos, then my sex toys stayed hidden in the bureau drawer.—Max

Finally, you may be sexual only with people you are not intimate with, finding it difficult to sustain a sexual relationship with someone you are very close to. You may feel that having sex with a confidant, lover, or partner is too dangerous.

I love my lover. We have been together seven years. I just can't sustain a sexual relationship with him. We have sex, and I feel horrible, afraid, and like I need to run away.—Debbie

I got to a point in my relationship where I didn't want to have sex at all anymore. The closer I got to my partner, the more she felt like family, and the more repulsed I became by sex. I took a break from sex, and then extended the break, but it wasn't helping. I wasn't getting closer to wanting sex or feeling better. I was just continuing to avoid dealing with combining intimacy and sex. The little girl in me just wanted to finally be loved for herself instead of for sex.—Melanie

What Are You Missing? The Costs of Aversion

While avoiding sex and your sexuality can seem like a good strategy for survival, the costs can be high. Staying away from erotic feelings, masturbation, and sex separates you from a powerful part of yourself. You lose a part of yourself that could feed vitality and energy into every aspect of your life. By avoiding sex, you lose a very deep means of connecting with yourself and others, not to mention the delight, joy, and fun that sex can bring you.

Perhaps more important, in avoiding sex, you communicate to yourself that you can't handle it, that the sexual abuse is bigger than you, and that sex is too much or too overwhelming for you. Sexual aversion keeps sex locked into the "Danger! Don't go there!" closet. While the sexual abuse *was* overwhelming and destructive and *did* control you at the time, your own sexuality and sexual expression are gifts that can help you heal now.

I want to collapse around sex. I feel small and it feels big.—Maria

Avoiding sex can feel like the best way to stay safe on a very visceral level. Sex was what was used to abuse you, so avoiding the weapon seems like a great strategy. But by avoiding your sexuality you can also trick yourself into thinking that you can avoid dealing with your history of sexual abuse. If you do not engage sexually, you may successfully avoid the triggers, flashbacks, and memories that sex can evoke. But you will have less and less room for you. The sexual abuse will continue to run the show.

Your own sexual energy is not too big for you now. You can learn how to embrace the sensations, the excitement, and, eventually, the delight of your sexuality. You can also build a capacity to be able to process the triggers that may emerge as you open to your own sexuality. Yes, this is difficult. But if you are not making your own choices about your sexuality, who is controlling it for you?

Your sexuality did not cause anyone to harm you. The abuse was the responsibility of those who harmed you. Your sexuality, no matter what they told you, is not at fault for your having been sexually abused as a child.

Sexual Compulsion: Sex As the Only Way

We are taught that sex is bad, and that if you are a woman and want a lot of sex—or even any sex at all—something must be wrong with you. I have heard many a survivor say that she was "acting out" when in fact she was expressing her self-defined sexuality. We have so few models for sexually empowered women that our sexual expression can be easily misinterpreted as sexual compulsion. As I talk about sexual compulsion, I am not referring to your fullest sexual expression. This is welcomed and encouraged. You may find that you are interested in sex more often than the culture deems "appropriate" for women. Again, sexual healing is about creating a sexuality based upon your own needs and desires, a sexuality of *your* choosing.

Some survivors go through a period in their sexual recovery during which sex may *feel* compulsive. This may be a phase of sexual healing or discovery that can be left alone and weathered. One woman describes her experience:

> *During one part of my healing, I was masturbating all the time. I was using fantasies of the abuse while I masturbated. I am so glad that my therapist just hung with me through it. She didn't judge me or tell me to get over it. Her sense was that I would ride it through, and I did. I learned a lot about my sexuality, sex toys, and phone sex. My sexual partner and I had a lot of phone sex that was really hot. I used the abuse fantasies until they weren't interesting anymore. Somehow all of that was a part of opening up my sexuality.* —Aurora

Sexual compulsion, on the other hand, is a real lack of choice. It is the inability to say "no"—or to even know how to make a conscious decision regarding sexual choices. You may be so checked out of your body that you only realize after the fact that you did not want the sex you just had. To truly consent, you need to be embodied and know how to say "yes," "no," and "maybe."

> *I had sex a lot. In the moment it seemed fine, but afterward, I would feel cheap, used, and dirty. I am just figuring out that I feel like this when I don't recognize my own wants and boundaries.* —Maggie

For some survivors who struggle with sexual compulsion, sex becomes one of the only means by which they feel worthy or able to interact with another person. If you struggle with this, you may be having sex to fill needs that are not necessarily sexual, such as needs for physical contact, intimacy, and self-worth. You may be having sex because you are hungry or because you need to be held. You may not realize that these needs can be met in other ways or that you are worthy of having your needs met at all.

I do not know that I am loved unless someone is having sex with me. Of course, once we are having sex, I think that is all they want me for. It's a catch-22.
—Hannah

Survivors of childhood sexual abuse can use sex as a way of avoiding feelings and staying dissociated. In this way, sex is used as a distraction or filler in an attempt to cope.

Sex became like alcohol for me. I couldn't cope with my life and with the abuse, so I'd go have sex instead. This made me feel better for a time, like a high, and then things would get worse. Sex was my enemy and my fix. It helped me get away from the pain, but acted out the pain at the same time.—Cindy

Incest and childhood sexual abuse destroy appropriate boundaries. Your physical, sexual, and emotional boundaries were shattered by abuse. To remain intact, some survivors attempt to live within their own destruction.

After awhile I figured it just didn't matter. My uncle and my dad were having sex with me, so that was what you do, right? I had sex with whoever.
—Stephanie

It got to a point in the abuse where I couldn't deal anymore. I thought, "So if this is what it's all about, fuck it! I'll play your game first." That is when I started being sexually aggressive with just about everyone in my life. I was known as the girl to go to in high school if you wanted to know anything about sex. Of course, I was also known as a slut. I derived this strange sense of power

from it all. My self-worth became completely entwined with people desiring me.
Essentially, I felt like I wasn't good for anything but sex.—Lourdes

You may be trying to work through the trauma by replaying it. This doesn't
heal the abuse, rather it keeps you stuck, doing the same thing over and over, and
not finding a way out.

What Are You Missing? The Costs of Compulsion

Perhaps the biggest cost of sexual compulsion is your own sexuality. While you
may look like a sexually expressive woman, sexual compulsion is not an expression of your own sexuality. While you may convince yourself that you want the
sex you are having, you are not really making choices based upon your own needs
and boundaries. Sexual compulsion runs you—you don't run it. An old survival
mechanism is still at play.

I thought I was just really sexually active. I notice though that mostly I am
spaced out when I am sexual. I don't think sex is bad, yet I am not really there.
Who is having sex when I am having sex? I'm not sure.—Carolyn

Another cost of sexual compulsion can be your self-esteem. When you have
sex that you don't really want, you undermine yourself. You trust yourself less
because you are not acting on your own behalf. This is exactly the behavior you
learned as a child. You are not bad for doing it, but it does not serve you any
longer.

In some ways the incest just goes on and on. Yes, I "consent" now with my
words, but I am saying "yes" to things I do not want. I just want to be close,
and I end up feeling so alone.—Cindy

Your physical health can be another cost of sexual compulsion. If you are
unable to say "no" to unwanted sex, you may also be unable to say "no" to unprotected sex. Having unprotected sex can put you at risk for sexually transmitted
diseases, including chlamydia, vaginal warts, herpes, and HIV. Whether you prefer numerous partners or serial monogamy, it is essential to practice safer sex using
condoms, dental dams, the female condom, latex gloves, or nonlatex substitutes.

Finally, through sexual compulsion you continue to have sex that it checked-out, keeping you out of your body and emotions. This keeps you out of your sexual healing, too.

Healing Self-Denial

Recovering from Sexual Aversion

When you focus on your recovery from sexual aversion, you propel your healing forward. As you do this, go slowly. If sex has been something you have avoided, you may be unfamiliar with your sexual desires and how to act and interact sexually.

Start by exploring the ways avoiding sex has served you. How has getting away from your sexuality protected or helped you? One workshop participant noted, "Staying away from sex helps me stay away from a huge sense of failure and loss. When I get sexual, I feel awful."

Next, explore what being sexual or turned on means to you. What do you associate with sex? Make a list entitled "Sex is…" or "Sex equals…" Your responses do not need to be logical or even make sense. Just look at what is tied up with sex for you. One survivor wrote, "Sex is hate, fear, and betrayal to me…No wonder I don't want to have it." Once you have made the list, try to determine which of these associations are inherent to sexual abuse and which of them are inherent to consensual sexual expression.

Consider what would be the worst possible outcome if you moved toward sex and your sexuality. What are you most afraid of? Then consider what would be the best possible outcome if you began to explore your sexuality.

Now, educate yourself. If you have been avoiding sex, you may be in need of information about your own sexuality and safer-sex practices. Seeking out this information in the form of books, magazines, audiotapes, and DVDs can give you models upon which to build a sexuality that works for you.

Sexual avoidance is really another form of dissociating or staying out of your body. Recovering from sexual avoidance means learning to tolerate the physical sensations and emotions that emerge when you are sexual. As you stay with the feelings and sensations, they will change, releasing the old trauma and letting you have your sexuality today. The pelvic rock and genital healing exercises in chapter 2 and the embodiment exercises in chapter 3 can help you learn to stay with and come to enjoy the feelings of sex and your sexuality.

You'll also find that masturbation is a wonderful tool for re-engaging with your sexual expression. Masturbation is not just about getting off. Through masturbation you can learn how to touch and love your body, discover your interests and desires, and learn about your own sensations and sexual energy. Chapter 5 is dedicated to the subject of self-loving.

When you open to your sexuality, you may experience a surge of energy that is unfamiliar to you. Your new sexual feelings may be unsettling. This is normal. In fact, it's progress! When you open to your own sexual desires and energy at a deeper level, you reorganize yourself.

> *Suddenly I felt sexual all the time. It was like I thought about sex, read about it, and felt it in my body twenty hours a day. I got nervous, worried I might become a nympho. This settled down after about a month. I had somehow opened up a door that had been long shut, and all the pressure needed to be released.—Sheila*

Recovering from Sexual Compulsion

What can you gain by healing your sexual compulsion? You gain your own sexuality on your own terms for possibly the first time in your life. This means that you get to choose whether you want to be sexual, with whom, when, where, and exactly what kind of sex you'd like to have. You can be fully in your body *and* be sexual. Healing compulsion also means you get to choose to *not* be sexual and still know you are loved and worthy. You get to take care of yourself based on your own needs and desires, instead of the needs and desires of another.

Just as with sexual avoidance, sexual compulsion has in some way benefited you. Do you know how sexual compulsion has served you? What does this compulsion do for you? What painful emotions does the compulsion help you avoid? What does it help you not face or feel? One survivor shared, "Having a lot of sex makes me feel powerful and keeps me from feeling the powerlessness I felt about what my granddad did."

What needs are you trying to fill when you have sex? Which of these needs are sexual and which are not? Are there particular abuse experiences that set you up to act compulsively?

What are you most afraid of in healing your sexual compulsion? What are you most looking forward to?

Now, educate yourself. If you have been acting compulsively with sex, you may not know when to be sexual and when not to, when sex takes care of you and when it doesn't. Talk to your friends, especially other survivors. What do they look for in sex? When do they say "no"? When do they say "yes"? You can also read about other folks' sexual expression and experiences. Read real-life stories instead of porn, as they will be more realistic.

Embodiment, Needs, and Boundaries

As with sexual avoidance, sexual compulsion is a way to remain out of your body. You may feel terrified or ashamed when you say "no" to sex or set a sexual boundary. Through recovery, you will learn how to feel the terror instead of distracting yourself from it. As you stay with the feelings and sensations, they will change, releasing the old trauma and letting you choose sex on terms that take care of you.

Chapter 3 on dissociation describes exercises to help you do this. Through recovery you will learn to be embodied when you are sexual and to have nonsexual needs met directly in nonsexual ways. "No" can become as easy to say as "yes." Chapter 7 is devoted to embodied consent. It features exercises on boundaries and the "yes," "no," and "maybe" of sex, which are useful in healing sexual compulsion.

While you are healing from sexual compulsion, you may want to consider taking some time off from sex altogether. You may choose to stop being sexual with others or to quit masturbating. A break from sex could be a week, a month, or a year. Choose a length of time that is realistic for you. In this time out from sex, see what comes up for you. What feelings or memories emerge? Who are you beyond sex?

Healing sexual compulsion gives you an opportunity to take care of yourself. As you stop using sex as a means to hold the hurt of the sexual abuse at bay, you also get the opportunity to truly heal and regain your life and your own sexuality.

Sexual Addiction Model

Some survivors find the addiction model of Twelve-Step programs useful in addressing sexual compulsion, while others have found it disempowering. Sex and Love Addicts Anonymous (SLAA) is a Twelve-Step program that deals specifically with sexual aversion and compulsion from an addiction model.

> I have done Twelve-Step recovery around my sexual stuff. Meetings are a place for me to get my bearings and support. They help me remember what is important to me, and I don't get judged if I mess up.—Lenore

> I was not addicted to love and sex, but rather acting out what happened to me. I was continuing to do what was done to me as a child. The more I dealt with my stepfather's abuse, the more I found boundaries and a kind of self-respect that let me start making choices sexually that took care of all of me. Calling it addiction, to me, makes me feel like something is wrong with me. This is my own body and my own energy that someone else harmed. I was surviving how I knew, and now healing is helping me find better and better options.—Kate

Choosing Celibacy

Choosing not to be sexual for periods of time can be useful in the journey of healing from child sexual abuse. If flashbacks to the sexual abuse are coming regularly, or if you feel like you hate sex, you might choose celibacy for a time. If you notice that you are having sex with yourself or a partner when you don't want to, try being intimate with yourself (or your partner) without being sexual.

> My partner and I are both survivors. I started dealing with my incest and ritual abuse four years into our relationship. Our sex life had actually been pretty good before that, but when all the memories came, I lost interest altogether. Sex

and abuse got all mixed up inside of me, and I just didn't want anything to do with it. We ended up taking a couple of breaks from sex that lasted between six and nine months each.—Jo

I kept having sex with my husband when I didn't want to. It wasn't him who was pushing me to do this. I would feel guilty about not being sexual with him and wanted to show him that I loved him and wanted him. This became really self-destructive and of course had an adverse affect on how I felt about him. Finally, I got the courage to negotiate three months off from sex… At the end of three months, we are going to check in to see how this is going and renegotiate from there.—Rona

Being celibate is a valid sexual choice. Celibacy can mean refraining from all overt sexual expression or being sexual with yourself while not having sex with others. You can be celibate for a period of time or as a lifelong choice. My concern about celibacy for survivors is that it can be used to mask an avoidance of the pain and hurt of the sexual abuse. If you are celibate because you don't know how to embrace your sexuality in a way that enhances and vitalizes your life, then celibacy is not a choice. When opting for celibacy, just make sure it is really a choice.

The End of Self-Denial

Ending self-denial does not mean you will become some hedonistic individual just out for herself. Ending self-denial, rather, means bringing yourself back into balance. It means respecting yourself deeply, which also allows you to respect others.

Sex Guide Exercises

1. Where do you fall on the scale of sexual aversion/sexual compulsion? List three instances when you avoided your sexuality and/or three instances when you had compulsive sex.
2. What emotions are you trying to manage through sexual compulsion or aversion?

chapter five

Sexual Response and Anatomy: Information Is Power

Childhood sexual abuse is about the worst way to learn about sex. Unfortunately, this is most likely the way that you were first exposed to sex—not what you would call a sex-positive sex education! Learning and relearning about sex is a lifelong endeavor for everyone, but it is especially so for survivors of sexual abuse. To help you along the way, this chapter is chock-full of information about your body and the sexual response cycle.

Where Did You Learn That?

I remember the first time a customer at Good Vibrations asked me where her clitoris was. I was both stunned and glad she had the courage to ask. Over time, I've learned that this was not an unusual situation. If no one teaches you or encourages you to learn about your own body, there is no reason you would know.

What do *you* know about your sexual anatomy? When did you first learn about your clitoris? Where did you get your information about sex and sexual arousal?

Studies show that most people learn about sex from their peers in their youth. So what we didn't learn from our abusers, we learned from a bunch of under-educated youth attempting to teach one another something they didn't know much about.

Other than your peers, the key source of information about your body and sexuality is the media. Movies, magazines, popular songs, and books tell us about ourselves and our bodies. Of course, some of these messages are more accurate and more positive than others.

You may have found your way to quality sex information, from recently published sex-positive books, or even from a supportive lover or friend. Congratulations! You are the rare breed. But if you have not had access to helpful sex information, please use this chapter as a friendly resource. It's hard to know what is up with your sexuality, much less successfully guide someone else toward your pleasure, if you do not know what happens to your body when you are turned on. Information is power, especially where sex is concerned!

Sex Information and Sexual Abuse

As a survivor, you were exposed to harmful negative information about your sexuality. You may have known a lot about sex, far more than was good for you, but the information was tarnished by the abuse—or just plain *wrong*. You learned about sex on the abuser's terms, not your own. You may have been taught how to gratify someone else sexually, without even knowing how to please yourself. This may have carried over into later consensual sexual relationships.

> *At thirteen I knew so much about sex and penises. My friends would ask me questions and couldn't believe how much I knew. I got this strange pride out of it, even though it was because of the sexual abuse that I knew all of that. Really, all I knew was how I was supposed to suck off my stepfather, how to give him what he demanded.—Laura*

> *I knew a lot about my boyfriend's body and hardly anything about my own. We had a very out-of-balance sex life. My pleasure was not really a part of it.—Cindy*

As a survivor, you may want to start all over in learning about sexual anatomy. Look at yourself, or a friend or partner, with curiosity. What is this thing, anyway? How does it feel?

So What Is That Thing? A Lesson in Sexual Anatomy

Female Sexual Anatomy

Let's begin with female anatomy. As you read this section, I encourage you to follow along—you can look at the illustration, and you can get out a mirror and check yourself out. As a woman, you do not get the opportunity to look at your genitalia often, because they are tucked in between your legs at an angle difficult to see unassisted. Although you may have been hurt in your genitals, there is nothing "wrong" with them. Your genitalia are as unique as the rest of you, a healthy and natural part of your body, just like your hand, your mind, and your face. Take a look. What do you see?

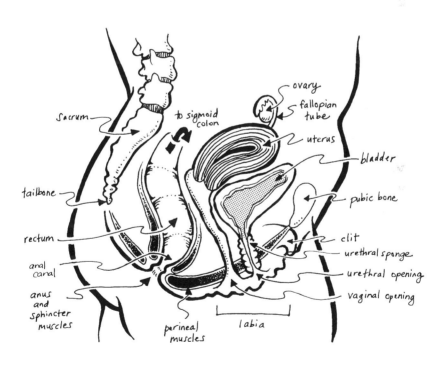

ILLUSTRATION 2. Female Anatomy

The entire genital region is called the vulva and includes the clitoris, the labia minora and labia majora, and the vagina. When you take a look at yourself in the mirror, you may first notice your labia majora and labia minora. These are your outer and inner vaginal lips, respectively. The labia majora have hair on them and are the same texture as your skin. The labia minora are hairless and made of mucous membrane, like the inside of your mouth. The inner lips come in all kinds of shapes and sizes. Some women's are symmetrical, while others are asymmetrical, one being much longer or larger than the other. Some women's inner lips fit within the outer lips, and others hang below the labia majora. What do yours look like? What color are they and what shape? Many survivors feel ashamed of their genitals because of sexual abuse. Your vulva deserves no shame. It is a perfectly healthy and important part of you body.

THE CLITORIS

With a mirror you can also see your clitoris and clitoral hood. These are tucked near the top of your labia minora. The clitoris is the most sensitive spot on the vulva. You can find it if you feel around in this area. The clitoral hood rides around the clitoris. You may find that your clitoris protrudes out of the clitoral hood or is tucked back within it. If you gently pull back the clitoral hood you'll see your clitoral glans.

Feminist health clinicians have helped to redefine the clitoris. We now know that the clitoris is not just the glans and shaft but encompasses a whole structure of erectile tissue, made up of nerves, spongy tissue, and blood vessels, that runs throughout the vulva. You may have seen illustrations in books like *A New View of a Woman's Body* or *Our Bodies, Ourselves,* which show the clitoral shaft splitting into two legs, called *crura,* that extend down through the labia minora around the vagina. If you press one of your labia minora between two fingers and rub slightly back and forth, you may be able to feel a sensitive ridge. This is one of the legs of the crura. If you feel upward from the head of the clit you can feel the clitoral shaft.

Clits comes in different sizes and sensitivities. Some women enjoy stimulation right on or near the clit, while others do not like to have their clit touched directly at all. Many women report that the clitoris is most sensitive halfway down the left-hand side. If you placed a clock over the clit with noon at the clitoral shaft and six nearer the vagina, this spot would be at three o'clock. Where is your clitoris most sensitive?

THE VAGINA

As you continue to explore yourself with the aid of the mirror, you will see the vaginal opening and the vagina. This too is made up of very pliable mucous membrane. The vagina itself is made up of folds of skin that are very expandable. When you are not sexually aroused, the walls of the vagina rest against one another. If you bear down while opening your inner labia with your fingers you can see the urethral opening (where urine comes out) just below the clitoris.

Different areas of the vagina feel differently when touched. The outer third of the vagina tends to be the most sensitive and responds to motion and movement. Deeper within the vagina, pressure and fullness tend to be more noticeable or satisfying.

At the back of the vagina is the cervix. This is a small, knoblike fleshy protrusion. A tiny opening in the cervix allows the passage of fluids in and out of the uterus. Menstrual blood flows out through the cervix, and sperm can swim in to impregnate a woman. The cervix dilates during childbirth to allow the baby to be passed out of the uterus through the vaginal canal into the world. Some women like to have their cervix pressed up against during sex. It can be a very particular and intense sensation. Try it for yourself and see what you think.

The vagina is a self-cleaning system with natural fluids and discharges. If your discharge is a color or smell that is unusual for you, or is accompanied by itching in the area, see a health care practitioner. Otherwise, your discharge is evidence of your cleansing system at work. Douches and other forms of cleansing within the vagina can destroy healthy bacteria. Oil-based lubricants are difficult for the vagina to cleanse and may cause an infection. Use water-based lubricants instead and avoid commercially prepared douches.

The vagina also self-lubricates when you are aroused. There are ducts and glands that produce lubrication along the walls of the vagina. Some women feel like they produce "too much" lubrication. Bring a towel with you on your sexual excursions; you may be ejaculating and not know it (see the following section for a discussion of female ejaculation). Your lubrication levels will change depending upon where you are in your cycle, and most women produce less lubrication as they age. If you don't produce enough moisture to make penetration comfortable, use a water-based lubricant.

THE G-SPOT

Also within the vaginal passage is the urethral sponge, or G-spot, a spongy conglomeration of blood vessels, erectile tissue and glands surrounding the urethra, the slim tube that carries urine from the bladder. The term G-spot was popularized by obstetrician and gynecologist Ernst Grafenberg, who wrote about the sensual properties of the urethra in 1950.

The G-spot is located along the front wall of the vaginal passage (closest to your public bone) and can be particularly sensitive to touch and especially sensitive to pressure. It is not really a "spot," but an area one to two inches in length. Again, bear down while opening your inner labia and you will see your G-spot. You can distinguish this tissue by its texture, which is rougher than the smooth walls of the rest of the vagina.

Women respond differently to G-spot stimulation. Some women find this touch intense and a great turn-on, while others find G-spot stimulation uncomfortable. Some women do not notice much difference in this area at all. Again, this is a time to explore, either alone or with a partner.

If you lie on your back, your partner can reach your G-spot by inserting two fingers into your vagina and making a "come hither" motion toward the front wall of your vagina. You can reach your own G-spot with fingers or a firm dildo. Dildos with a ridged area or a curve or bend in the shaft can be particularly good G-spot stimulators. Once you are sexually aroused, your G-spot can also be reached by placing pressure on the abdomen just above the pubic bone and pressing down toward the vaginal opening.

Some women ejaculate with G-spot stimulation. The ejaculate is watery in substance and is sometimes mistaken for urine. Within the spongy material of the urethra are the paraurethral glands, which are thought to be the origin of the G-spot ejaculate. The theory is that with pressure and stimulation, these glands produce the fluid that is released as ejaculate; just as in men, the ejaculate comes through the urethra. Although there is still some debate as to the exact origin of the ejaculate, the majority of studies have found the fluid chemically distinct from urine. Not all women seem to ejaculate with G-spot stimulation, however. More information about stimulating the G-spot can be found in chapter 10.

Male Sexual Anatomy

Men's sexual anatomy is not drastically different from women's, when you get right down to it. All fetuses are initially female in their genitalia. Between nine and twelve weeks, the genitalia begin to differentiate. What becomes the clitoris in the female becomes the glans of the penis in the male. While ovaries develop in females, the testes develop in males. The components of male and female sexual anatomy are very similar; they are just arranged differently.

Male sexual anatomy is made up of the penis, scrotum, and testicles, the seminal vesicle, and the prostate gland. The penis and the scrotum, which contains the testicles (the "balls," in slang), are the most obvious parts of male sexual anatomy. Let's start with these.

THE PENIS AND BALLS

The penis is made up of spongy erectile tissue and blood vessels. These tissues are organized into two long cylinders called the corpus cavernosa. When a man is sexually aroused, blood flows into these cylinders, filling the spongy tissues. They expand as they fill with blood, compressing shut the veins that carry blood out of the penis, thus creating an erection, or hard-on.

The urethra, the tube through which urine and semen pass, runs along the bottom of the penis to the urethral opening at the tip. It is surrounded by a cylinder of spongy tissue called the corpus spongiosum.

The head of the penis is also called the glans. This is the most sensitive part of the penis. The base of the head is called the coronal ridge and is analogous to the clitoris in the woman. The nerves here are not as densely concentrated as the clitoral nerves, however, and therefore the area is not as sensitive. The head of the penis can usually stand more pressure and stimulation than the clitoral glans. The frenulum, a piece of skin on the underside of the coronal ridge between the shaft of the penis and the glans, is also packed with nerves and sensitive for many men.

The skin covering the penis slides easily back and forth. All men are born with a foreskin, a retractable skin, which covers the glans. When men are circumcised, this skin is cut off, exposing the head. Men with foreskins tend to be more sensitive around the head of the penis than circumcised men.

The penis has been a frightening piece of male anatomy for many survivors of child sexual abuse. Begin to demystify it for yourself by learning about it in a nonabusive setting. You can look at human anatomy books with pictures. If you have a male partner, you can ask to look at his penis in a nonaroused state. Try to

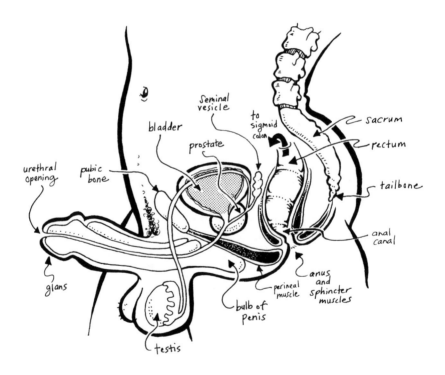

ILLUSTRATION 3. Male Anatomy

consider the penis as a neutral part of a man's whole body. It is his person, not his penis, that decides how it will be used. Your perpetrators made very destructive choices.

If learning more about male sexual anatomy is upsetting for you, this may be a place to work through those triggers (for help, see chapter 11). Even if you do not interact sexually with men, freeing yourself from the fear of male sexuality will greatly benefit you. It can give you freedom in your relationship to your own body and sexuality, and in your relationship to men in general. Holding emotional trauma connected to the anatomy of half of the world's population requires energy that you can use more creatively in enjoying your life.

"Balls" is slang for the scrotum and testicles. The scrotum is the skin surrounding the testicles, two glands that produce both sperm and testosterone. The testicles range from the size of a grape to that of an egg. One usually hangs lower than the other, and they contract up closer to the body when a man is cold or aroused.

The Prostate Gland

The prostate gland is an internal organ located behind the pubic bone in front of the bladder. The urethra passes from the bladder through the prostate into the penis. This gland produces seminal fluids. I mention it because many men find prostate stimulation very pleasurable. Like G-spot stimulation in women, prostate stimulation may be too intense or painful for some. The prostate can be reached by inserting a finger or toy about three inches into the anus and pressing toward the front of the body. It is that old "come hither" motion again. If you are planning to play with your partner's prostate, be sure to use a water-based lubricant, as the anus is not self-lubricating.

Female and Male Bodies

The PC Muscle

The pubococcygeus muscle, or the PC muscle for short, runs from the pubic bone to the tailbone, surrounding the genitals in a figure eight. This is the muscle you squeeze to stop the flow of urine. It is also the muscle that involuntarily contracts with orgasm. Your PC muscle is important to your health and sexual satisfaction. A healthy and well-exercised PC muscle can keep you from being incontinent, increase your orgasmic pleasure, and help you be more embodied in your pelvis and genitals. You can also contract this muscle at will to play with your sexual pleasure.

Exercising this muscle is easy. Practice contracting the PC muscle by squeezing your genitals and anus inward ten times. Then bear down, pushing them outward ten times. Do this three time a day. These exercises are referred to as kegels. Doing your kegels will keep these muscles in good condition and increase your awareness of your genitals.

> Doing kegels stirred up all kinds of anger for me initially. I would want to growl and kick. I guess it stirred up the stuff that was in my pelvis from the abuse. —Jackie

> Exercising my PC muscle has given me more of a sense of control over my own genitals. It made them feel less separate from me. I realized that they were mine and I could move them and do something with them. It wasn't just that things got done to them.—Kate

BREASTS

Both women and men can experience sexual pleasure in their breasts. When sexually aroused, many people's nipples respond by becoming erect or hard. Some folks enjoy intense pressure and sensation on their nipples, while others like a softer touch or caress.

Many survivors report not having a lot of sensation in their breasts or nipples. If this is the case for you, you may be experiencing some numbing of sensation due to the abuse. Or, this may just be the way your body responds. If you want to explore this, bring your focus to your breasts. Breathe into your breasts. Lay your hands over your breasts. Feel the weight of your hands. What is there? Try touching your breasts with more or less pressure and creating different sensations. Aroused nipples can actually take quite a lot of pressure. Try pinching or squeezing harder (or ask your partner to do so). Try this on the nipple, or grab below the nipple on the areola. By practicing this, you may increase your sensitivity. You may also discover trauma related to your breasts.

I have very little sensation in my breasts. I think I can't feel them because of the incest. When my husband touches them, I can't feel it and I start to dissociate.—Sally

ANAL EROTICISM

The anus carries a lot of social taboo when it comes to sexual pleasure. Many folks think of the anus as dirty or painful and hold a lot of tension there. Whether or not you include anal eroticism in your sex life, learning to relax the anus enhances your health and allows for more sensation throughout the genital area.

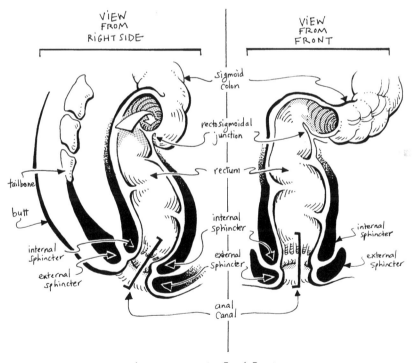

ILLUSTRATION 4. Anal Anatomy

Just like the vulva and penis, the anus engorges with blood when sexually aroused and shares in the muscle contractions of orgasm.

The anal opening is controlled by two rings of muscles called the sphincters. You can learn to relax and contract the external sphincter at will; the internal sphincter operates involuntarily, like blinking. Beyond these muscles is the rectum, an expandable canal six to nine inches in length, which is lined with a very soft tissue. This tissue is not as durable as vaginal tissue, and microscopic tears can happen during penetration. This makes practicing safer sex when engaging in anal eroticism all the more important.

The rectum ends in an S-shaped curve called the rectosigmoidal junction. Beyond this point is the sigmoid colon and the large intestine. Feces are stored on the intestine side of this S-curve. When you feel that you have to defecate, you are feeling pressure on the rectosigmoidal junction. Feces only pass through the rectum; they are not stored there. There are usually few traces left behind.

Unlike the vaginal canal, the anus leads directly into the internal organs of the body. If you are interested in using toys for anal penetration, it is vital to choose toys that have an expanded or flanged base that will not slip up into the rectum and potentially the large intestine. Lubricant is a *must* for anal penetration. More information on anal sex, cleanliness, lubrication, and anal penetration can be found in chapters 9 and 10 on oral sex and penetration.

Finally, the soft piece of skin between the vagina and anus in women, or between the scrotum and anus in men, is called the perineum. This is another area where you can enjoy pressure and touch.

Checking In

Take a minute to check in with yourself. How are you doing reading about sex and sexual anatomy? What are you feeling in your body? What are your automatic thoughts as you read through this chapter? Take a breath and a break, if need be.

Sexual Response Cycle

Your body goes through many physiological changes when sexually aroused and during orgasm. Masters and Johnson popularized the phrase "sexual response cycle" by somewhat arbitrarily organizing female and male physiological sexual responses into four phases: excitement, plateau, orgasm, and resolution.

As per their definition, the excitement phase involves a general increase in body temperature, heart rate, and blood flow. The increased blood flow enlarges the lips, breasts, and genitals. Usually the body becomes more sensitive to stimulation and less sensitive to pain.

In the plateau stage, the blood flow and body temperature continue to increase. In women, the labia and clitoris enlarge and the uterus lifts, creating a ballooning effect in the vagina. The vagina also lubricates. In men, the increased blood flow creates an erection, and the testes and scrotum contract and lift. Men can also excrete a fluid called "pre-come." Both women and men may experience erections in the nipples.

In the Masters and Johnson model, orgasm is the next stage. Orgasm is defined as a release of the sexual buildup in a series of muscular contractions. Orgasm releases the increased blood from the genital tissues. After orgasm comes resolution, when the body returns to a nonaroused state. The body cools, the heart rate drops again, and the blood flows out of the breasts and genitals, returning them to their at-rest state.

I offer this model as a description of the physiological changes that occur during sexual arousal. This is not a prescription for how sexual arousal *should* go or even *does* go; it is just one interpretation of how it might go. Your experience may sometimes match this model and other times not.

Other sexologists have categorized the stages of sexual arousal differently, trying to account for the more subjective experiences and social and cultural influences involved in sexual response. Some suggest including desire as a stage of sexual response. Another begins her model with willingness. In *The Good Vibrations Guide to Sex*, Cathy Winks and Anne Semans speak of the overall fluidity of sexual response: "One can move from arousal to desire, from excitement to indifference, from boredom to passion, from orgasm to arousal and back again."

I want to note particularly for survivors that with sexual stimulation this physiological response of arousal occurs whether or not the sex is consensual. So many survivors blame themselves or hate their bodies because they got aroused during the abuse. This response is involuntary. It is what your body does when stimulated. Physical pleasure makes the abuse all the more confusing. But remember that the fact that you became aroused does not mean you wanted to be abused, that the abuse was your fault, or that your body betrayed you.

Orgasm

An orgasm is one of those experiences that no one seems to exactly know how to describe. I have heard people say, "You'll know when you have one," which may be true but is not very helpful. Physiologically, an orgasm is an involuntary contraction of the muscles in the pelvic region, and the lower third of the vagina, that results from sexual stimulation.

Some women speak about a clitoral orgasm as distinct from a vaginal orgasm. Sometimes an orgasm is very localized around the clit or vagina, and other times it can be spread over the entire body. There is still much to be known about women's sexuality, and even authoritative physiological texts disagree.

There are numerous books available on the subject of the female orgasm and techniques you can try to explore and enhance your orgasms. Again, the more you are able to relax and embody your pelvis and genitals, the more sensation you will have. Focusing your attention on your sensations and breathing down into your pelvis and genitals will help you increase your pleasure.

Orgasm and Ejaculation

Contrary to popular belief, ejaculation and orgasm are separate physiological functions controlled by different nerve groups in the spine. This is true for both men and women. Although many people experience them simultaneously, neither G-spot ejaculation in women nor ejaculation in men necessarily correspond to an orgasm. One can learn to separate these functions with practice.

Multiple Orgasms

Yup, multiple orgasms are possible. Multiple orgasms are a series of orgasms, one following the next. Most of the time people experience a short rest moment in between orgasms and then continue onto the next. Some folks also talk about a continuous or extended orgasm. Annie Sprinkle teaches the one-hour orgasm in *The Sluts and Goddesses Video Workshop*. Both multiple orgasms and extended orgasms are learnable through practice. The first step is learning to be with the intensity of continuing stimulation once you have had an orgasm. Then, breathing deeply and rocking your pelvis, combined with stimulation that works for you, will show you the way.

Are You Preorgasmic?

Some women have never experienced an orgasm. Sex educators use the term preorgasmic to describe this state. We call it "preorgasmic" because we assume that women can learn to orgasm. Many women who are preorgasmic have not experienced the type of stimulation that works for their anatomy.

The majority of women need direct clitoral stimulation to orgasm. Most women need continuous, steady, and sometimes rapid stimulation to come. Vibrators can be very useful when learning to orgasm. They create a faster and more intense stimulation than most people can muster with their fingers and also let you explore a variety of sensations.

Being preorgasmic can be linked to sexual trauma. You may carry a lot of tension in your pelvis and genitals, which makes it difficult to relax enough to orgasm. Most people think of orgasm as a tensing of the muscles, but the more you can relax, the better, since it can be difficult for the muscles to go from a very contracted state into an even more contracted state for orgasm. The more you breathe and relax your pelvic muscles, the easier it is to orgasm.

I can't orgasm. I get really tight through my pelvis and seem on the verge forever. I just can't get over the top.—Maria

Some survivors also feel shame, guilt, or other emotions that are a part of the sexual trauma connected to orgasm. You may want to avoid orgasm to avoid these feelings. Use the practices in chapter 11 to assist you in working through these triggers and held trauma.

If you are preorgasmic, I encourage you to explore orgasm on your own—not just with a partner—so that you can take your time without pressure or expectations. Most important, breathe as you begin to touch yourself. Notice when you want to hold your breath and relax again. Breathe down into your pelvis as if you could nourish the pelvic cavity and your genitals with oxygen. Allow yourself to move your hips. Do not hold yourself still; rock your hips forward and back, side to side, and around in a small circle. You may feel silly at first, but keep going. This is you getting to know *you*.

I encourage you to invest in a vibrator. You can try placing the vibrator directly on different places around your clit, vagina, perineum, and anus. Where are you the most sensitive? Where do you like more pressure and where less? Where is the most sensitive spot on your clit? If a vibrator is too intense initially, place a towel between you and it, or place the vibrator on the outside of your outer labia, letting the vibration pass through the folds of skin to the clitoris. Or try the vibrator on the back of your hand as you touch your clit with your fingers. As you find your most sensitive spots, stay with the feeling, and continue to breathe and rock. Keep bringing your attention into your body and genitals. Feel yourself. Be inside of yourself and your sensations. Make sure your internal conversation supports what you are doing rather than distracts you. Tell yourself that being turned on is great, that it is okay to relax and to have sexual pleasure. Tell yourself something sexy!

Again, you may find that working with your orgasm brings up emotions and images related to the sexual abuse. Our bodies can act as storage tanks for pieces of the abuse that we have not yet been able to fully feel or process. The emergence of these pieces of the past is part of your healing process. Your body is releasing trauma associated with, or held in, this part of your body. Go into and through these emotions, triggers, and memories. You may cry, get angry, or shake. Don't worry. This is a normal part of the healing process.

This Is Taking Too Long

While not preorgasmic, some women feel like it takes them too long to come to orgasm. But "too long" is relative. My first question would be, "Too long by whose standards?"

When we go to the movies, we see instantaneous sex. Two people meet, get turned on, make love, come simultaneously, and *voila*! It is over. Sex and orgasm are not like that in real life. A more typical sexual encounter involves talking, rearranging your bodies a number of times, laughing, at least one awkward moment, farting or trying not to, and so on. Sorry to burst your bubble, but my intent is to normalize sex. Yes, sex can be profound and powerful, just as other parts of our lives can be, but sex is also a normal aspect of the human experience. We bring the rest of our humanness with us when we are sexual.

So, back to orgasm taking "too long." What you mean by too long? Is ten minutes too long? Is half an hour? What if you focused on reaching orgasm for three hours? What if your partner focused on your pleasure for three hours? How would that be? I find that most people's time expectations for orgasm are too brief, particularly for women. What if you let yourself take more time than you are comfortable with? Try it.

If you would like to have the option of reaching orgasm more quickly, you can try using a vibrator; the intense stimulation can bring you to orgasm faster. The breathing and movement techniques described above will also help. Usually, tension in the pelvis and genitals delays orgasm. Move, relax, and breathe. If your partner is not touching you in a way that works, let her or him know that. Communicate what you like and show your partner how to do it. You'll both be happier in the long run.

Last, if you feel like you come to the edge but cannot go over it, try shifting your internal focus. If you are focused on your clitoris, open up your focus to include the sensations throughout your pelvis and throughout the rest of your body. Often this can relax you enough to allow you to orgasm.

Gynecological Issues

Incest and childhood sexual abuse can cause a number of gynecological problems. Some survivors experience external or internal scarring from the abuse. Others have chronic yeast infections or sexually transmitted diseases from the abuse. Still others have menstrual irregularities and pelvic or genital pain. If you have any chronic infections, menstrual difficulties, pain, or other concerns, please see a gynecologist. Eastern medicine, acupuncture, has shown to be very successful with gynecological issues as well. Before you take on the emotional angle of this work, please see a health practitioner to take care of any medical issues you may have.

> *I have had chronic yeast infections since I was seven and my stepfather started molesting me.—Kate*

What I see with many survivors is a chronic holding or tension throughout the pelvis. Tensing and pulling away from abuse and intrusion is a natural response. It is an attempt to protect yourself and to get away. This tension can become habitual or chronic and cause other problems. I have seen survivors with ongoing yeast infections and medically unexplained pains that correlated to the ways they were abused.

Chronic tension or holding in the pelvis causes a constriction of blood flow through the area. Held tension and trauma in the body can also decrease your sensations. Some people talk about trauma as energy blocked or trapped in the pelvis. Put your attention into the sensations in your pelvis and ask yourself the following questions: What sensations can I feel in my pelvis and genitals? Are the sensations warm or cool? Does my pelvis feel blank or void? Do I feel any streaming or movement? What images or colors come to mind as I focus there? Does my pelvis feel connected to my legs? To my torso?

> *When I first started focusing on recovering my sexuality, my vagina and pelvis felt like stone. I would get an image of dried, cracked earth that nothing could grow in. I imagined watering it, loosening it, and making it more flexible. The more I moved and tried to feel myself there, the more I touched myself and tried to become friends with me again, the more that image changed.—Stephanie*

Your Body

Many survivors have a difficult relationship with their bodies. You may struggle with body hate, feeling that your body has betrayed you or that your body is an unsafe place to live. Having a body at all may be a problem for you. You may struggle with anorexia or bulimia, or feel you are over- or underweight. Many survivors use food a means of coping with their emotions, while others have a difficult time feeding themselves at all. Since your body was touched or used during the abuse, a difficult relationship with your body is often one of the lasting effects.

Sometimes survivors do not like their bodies because the body is where pain lives. Getting in touch with your body can also mean attending to the trauma that is still held there.

I always felt like my body was his. It wasn't mine. It had betrayed me and now it was his ally and my enemy.—Maggie

As you consider your relationship with your body, especially your sexual body, examine who taught you about your body. Where did you pick up this information? What makes this opinion so valid?

I know that our relationships with our bodies run very deep. It is not like you can say, "Oh, okay, I decided I want to believe something different from what I was taught, so now I feel differently." Changing your relationship with your body and sexuality is a multilevel process. First, you must look at what you do believe and who you learned that from. Is this who you want to have say over your relationship to your own body? If you were to write the script of your relationship to your body, what would it say?

Next come the practices to support this. What can you say to yourself that supports the relationship you want to build with your body? What is a small step in that direction? A medium and a big step? You might start by writing down the script you'd like hold as your truth. Then tell one trusted friend that new story. Tape it to your bathroom mirror so that you see it and read it daily. Let other people in your life know that this is the new relationship with your body you are creating. Ask them to see you in this new light.

The same somatic practices that helped you discover a sense of internal safety (see chapter 1) will help you create a new, more loving relationship with your body. Martial arts, yoga, dance, sports, meditation, and other embodiment practices that bring your attention to the sensations in your body are also powerful allies in helping you release the trauma that has supported your negative relationship with your body. You may need to walk through shame and guilt, and begin to place your rage and anger with your perpetrators instead of internalizing it as self-blame. You may need to face the grief of loss and betrayal that hating your body keeps you from feeling. What is it that you are most afraid to let yourself feel? If you were to build an empowering relationship with your body—including your sexual body— what emotions would come up? How can you begin to move toward your feelings?

> *Being in my own body and liking me there is one of the hardest parts of my recovery. I hate it when people say "just love your body." That sounds so trite in comparison to what I am dealing with in here. I am taking a step at a time in accepting me, and finding small bits of pleasure in my body. That part is cool.—Danielle*

The Body Hug

This exercise can greatly assist you in learning to know, accept, and even like those parts of your body you have learned to hate. Practice this any place on your body where you feel targeted, were abused, or dislike your body.

Find a calm place to sit or lie down. Relax and deepen your breathing, expanding your belly and your chest. As you lie there, bring your attention into your hands. You can rub them together to warm them and bring energy into them. Put love and acceptance into your hands. To do this you can think of someone or something you love and feel warmth for. Then place your hands on whatever part of your body you have chosen to work with. Gently let your hands rest there, or stroke that part of you. Bring loving-kindness into that part of you.

Your mind will probably go wild, ticking off all the things you feel are wrong with that part of your body. You are too fat—look at that!—you are too skinny, you've got stretch marks, you sag, your skin is bad...

Write these down if you need to. What are the feelings underneath all that chatter? What memories are stirred in this part of your body? Note these, then return to your breathing and your accepting touch. Keep coming back to the warmth and care in your hands. Try this for five minutes.

You can now develop a powerful relationship with your body, with living in your own skin. You can learn to appreciate what was perhaps never appreciated, to respect yourself in the ways you were not respected.

Sex Guide Exercises

1. What three life experiences most informed your relationship with your body and sexual body? These may be positive or negative influences. Consider family and community, abuse, social and cultural influences, media, sports or athletics, art and performance.

2. What part of your body do you have a difficult relationship with? Your stomach, breasts, hips, thighs? Get out paper and crayons or markers and draw that part of your body. It doesn't need to be a realistic rendition; just draw *your* impression of that part of your body. What does the image have to communicate to you? What does that part of your body need or want?

    I did this exercise with a woman who drew her genitals and pelvic region. Large parts of the initial drawing were black, squiggly lines marking up the page. Other parts of the drawing were nearly blank, as if this part of her body did not exist. As we worked, over time, she continued to draw images of her pelvic region. As she faced the trauma to this region of her body and welcomed her pelvis back into her life, the images changed. Bright colors started showing up in the drawings, and the area became more contained, less chaotic. The later drawings were both calm and fiery, very vibrant.

3. Get a mirror, and find a comfortable place and a time when you won't be interrupted. Look at your genitals. What do they look like? Identify your labia, clitoris and clitoral hood, vaginal opening, perineum, and anus.

4. What else might you like to learn about your own body, sexual response cycle, or capacity for orgasm? Choose one thing and start exploring.

chapter six

Masturbation and Self-Healing

Self-Loving

Masturbation is touching yourself sensually or sexually—regardless of whether or not you have an orgasm. Masturbation is good for lots of things. By touching yourself, you can learn what turns you on and what leaves you cold. Not only will this enhance your sexual enjoyment, it is the most important information you can give to a lover.

> *Masturbation is the center of my sexuality now. I have learned that I turn myself on, that I am responsible for my own pleasure. This has been so liberating for me.—Anna*

Masturbation is good for your health, too. Studies show that masturbation reduces stress and helps you relax. Also, regular use of your PC muscle keeps it in shape, increasing orgasmic pleasure, supporting childbirth, preventing incontinence, and in some cases reducing menstrual cramps.

Through masturbation you can explore your sexual responses, play with your fantasies, try out sex toys and safer-sex gear, expand your erotic repertoire, and build a positive relationship to own body and sexuality. You can have fun getting off, too!

Any trigger that gets set off with a partner will also show up in masturbation. When you masturbate, you can practice handling these triggers. Masturbation will help you learn in your own bed, through your own experiences, that your sexuality is yours, and that you are not "damaged" or "bad."

A Bad Rap

Masturbation has gotten a bad rap; it has been cited as the cause of insanity, blindness, impotence, hysteria, and other unrelated mental and physical symptoms. As recently as 1995, Dr. Joycelan Elders was asked to resign from her position as U.S. Surgeon General because she recommended masturbation as a form of safer sex.

Most of us have been taught from an early age that touching ourselves "down there" is bad. We are shamed out of self-exploration. We inherit a sex-negative view of masturbation that moves us away from a sense of pleasure in our own bodies.

It seems utterly sick to me that I was not supposed to touch myself sexually, but my father was allowed to do whatever he wanted to. Shouldn't that be the other way around?—Liz

Yet, nearly everyone masturbates. The Kinsey Institute reported in 1990 that 94 percent of men and 71 percent of women masturbate to orgasm. Masturbation is a healthy part of sexual development in children and a healthy part of sexual expression for adults. Fetuses have been noted to have erections and genital swelling in the womb, and infants discover that touching their genitals feels good. By two most toddlers are masturbating, and as they age, they become curious about others' bodies. All of this is part of a child's natural development.

What better way to develop sexually than to masturbate? Masturbation gives you a full range of choices about your own body and pleasure, and it puts your sexuality back into your own hands.

Your Keystone to Healing

Having sex with yourself is your most powerful recovery tool. Through masturbation you can practice all the components of sexual healing and recovery. You can practice being embodied, feeling your body move and come alive. You can work through triggers and face intrusive memories. You can discover where your body is frozen or unfeeling as a result of the abuse. And through masturbation you can practice being present during sex.

> I didn't really know how to masturbate. I just knew I wasn't suppose to do it. Once I finally learned it was okay, I realized that this was the best way for me to learn about my sexuality on my own terms.—Roslyn

> I have worked through a lot of my abuse through masturbating and fantasy. I re-created abuselike scenes in my fantasies, having them turn out differently than the abuse did.—Marie

Masturbation can help you explore the ways that sexual abuse has affected your sexuality and sexual expression. You don't have to wait for partner sex to bring your emotional responses and triggers to the foreground. When you masturbate, you'll find out *exactly* where the effects of incest and molestation landed in your body, emotions, and thinking.

> I learned to slow down and not just go for the orgasm masturbating. As I began to pay closer attention, I saw the entire cycle of my sexual "stuckness." I begin to get sexually aroused, begin to feel excited, and then get a wave of shame: "I am not supposed to be doing this." I keep masturbating, and the next wave is guilt: "See, I do like it, so I did deserve the abuse." If I can keep breathing and touching myself, the grief and the sadness under the guilt and shame come up. Usually then I cry. I get farther each time, though. I used to stop at the shame, and just shut down. I feel like now I am unpacking that guilt and shame from on top of my sexuality and feeling the deeper levels. I am freeing myself up. —Stephanie

I would start to masturbate and then feel a surge of guilt. It seemed that as soon as I felt pleasure I felt guilt. This was all about the incest.—Rosa

If the sexual abuse affected you in a way that makes you fear sex, masturbation offers you a slow and safe way to discover your sexual self amid the wreckage of abuse. Masturbation can assist you in moving from sexual repression to sexual expression.

I hated all sex. Masturbation didn't even cross my mind. I was relieved when my husband didn't want to have sex. Only after our divorce did I feel safe enough to wonder about my sexuality. A girlfriend gave me a book on sex that talked about masturbation as something healthy. I tried it. That was really the beginning of my healing.—Evelyn

If you have attempted to deal with the trauma of sexual abuse by becoming compulsive sexually, masturbation will help you to learn about boundaries and to heal the pain that drives the compulsion. Here you can practice paying attention to those feelings that say "stop here," or "I'd like to pause here." Stop when you feel those impulses. What is it like to feel and act on your own boundaries?

I had sex with everyone. I thought that being sexual would get me acceptance, would allow me to finally fit in. I kept doing this after I knew it was only hurting me. It is only recently that I have stopped. Now I'm trying to find my own likes and dislikes, my own boundaries. Being sexual with myself is helping me do that.—Lenore

Want to stretch the envelope of your sexual expression? In masturbating you can try out what would be too scary with a sexual partner. You'll discover parts of your sexuality that were hidden under the rubble of incest and molestation. As you become more confident in your self-exploration, you will be better equipped to communicate your desires to a sexual partner.

But I Don't Want to Masturbate

For some survivors, masturbation is linked to sexual abuse. One survivor I worked with was found masturbating by her grandfather; this was used as the justification for molesting her. Her enjoyment of masturbation "proved" that she "wanted" it.

> *He came into my room when I was six. I was touching myself and smelling my hand. I liked the smell of my vagina. This was the first time he molested me. He said girls who like that are dirty whores, and he'd just treat me like one too.*—Daren

Some survivors don't want to masturbate at all. Some women have cultural or religious reasons for not wanting to masturbate; others just don't like it. Healing is all about consent and choice. If you don't want to masturbate, you don't have to.

But before you decide not to masturbate, I encourage you to explore these questions: What emotions come up when you masturbate or even imagine masturbating? Do you experience self-blame, shame, guilt, rage, or grief? Is this also how you feel about the abuse? Is this how you feel about sex in general? Make a list of all the reasons you don't want to masturbate. Are you making your own choice, or is the abuse deciding for you?

Feelings and Triggers

For many survivors, masturbating brings up traumatic emotions. You might feel like your emotions will overwhelm you. The odd thing about healing trauma is that you may feel like you are going to die, or that you will be swallowed whole by your emotions, but you won't. As you let yourself experience these emotions, your tolerance for feeling them will increase. You will feel them and then they will pass. Feeling emotions is a large part of healing them.

> *I'm too triggered by sex to even masturbate. I feel so ashamed and dirty. I don't want to do to myself what my mom did to me.*—Carolyn

When I masturbate I become obsessed with coming. I get uptight and manic. I want to come and then get out of there.—Naomi

For many survivors, feeling sexual pleasure brings up shame about having experienced sexual pleasure during the sexual abuse. Many survivors were purposefully brought to orgasm during the abuse.

I get turned on, I feel guilty. I get turned on, I feel guilty. It is like this predictable cycle. What I know now, though, is that if I keep going through the guilt to the other side, it doesn't last. I feel turned on again. I am getting to really know that it is okay for me to be turned on.—Liz

Rage and grief are also common emotions for survivors when masturbating. You might feel these emotions every time you get turned on. If you feel like crying or raging during masturbation, go ahead. What are you grieving about? What are you angry about? Grieve for your losses. Get angry at your abusers. Hold yourself tenderly through this.

Sometimes when I masturbate, if I get really into it I get so angry I want to kick something.—Pam

I cry when I masturbate. I cry when I have an orgasm.—Danielle

Intrusive memories or images of the abuse may surface when you masturbate, too.

Lots of my memories have come while masturbating. I guess I feel safer being alone and relaxed, and they tend to come up.—Debbie

Once and for all I wanted to kick my father out of my head while I was masturbating. There he'd be again, his face and his dick. One time I stood up and yelled at him. I said, "That's it, get the hell out of here, you are not allowed here anymore. Get out!" He only came back once more after that, with much less force. Now I can intercept him at the door with a clear "no."—Janet

As you masturbate you can expect at some point to face deep emotions or triggers from the abuse. Know when this happens that you are healing. In the following chapters, you will find lots of tools and options for working with your triggers and emotions that emerge during masturbation and partner sex.

Now, on to the fun part!

Five Steps to Great Masturbation

You would think that masturbation would be self-explanatory, but, like anything else, it is a learned skill. There is an art to masturbation, and there are some basic moves that can make it more satisfying.

1. Breathe and Relax

As you touch yourself erotically, breathe. If you are touching your breasts or your belly, breathe into that area of your body. The breath helps you to be aware of the feelings and sensations there. When you are touching your vulva or clit, bring your breath all the way down into your pelvis. Imagine that you can breathe right into your vulva. Breathing helps to keep your body relaxed and uncontracted, thus letting you experience more feeling, sensation, and awareness of what is happening for you.

Breathing is particularly important for survivors. When we are afraid, we tighten our muscles and stop breathing. As you know, this is a great system for self-protection and helps numb sensation. For many survivors, this automatic response is still hooked up to being sexual or to masturbating. You may notice when you are sexual that you want to hold your breath or hold your muscles tight.

My jaws get incredibly tight when I masturbate. It's like I get tighter as I get turned on.—Marianne

When you catch yourself getting tense, breathe and relax. Bring your attention back to the feelings in your body.

When you breathe and relax your body while you masturbate, you are communicating something new to your body—that it is safe to feel sexually turned on, that it is fine to get off and to enjoy pleasure. Relaxation communicates safety to your body on a very deep level.

When I speak of relaxation, I do not mean becoming passive or comatose. You can relax and be actively engaged at the same time. You can still have an orgasm when you are relaxed; in fact, your orgasms will be more intense.

2. Move Your Body

The second important practice in masturbating is to move your body. Move your hips, rock your pelvis, let your back arch and press, move your arms, legs, and head. Let your body move and express your sensations and feelings. This may be embarrassing at first, but it is invaluable to your sexual pleasure and healing.

Moving also assists you in not freezing up your body; and it increases the sensations and allows them to spread throughout your body. If you are preorgasmic, moving can assist you in freeing up your orgasm.

Moving can also stir up body memories. Because many of us were held down or pinned during the abuse, moving your body can begin to loosen these held memories. Moving tells your body that you have the say-so now, that you are no longer frozen or paralyzed. You can act on your own behalf.

> I am at the point now where I love to move. I love to move with my honey and with just me. It makes me feel like I am free.—Jennifer

3. Make Some Noise

Making noise is the third great masturbation tool. You can start with breathing heavily, making noise on your exhalation. Let yourself "ooh" and "aahhh." Groaning and moaning is good for you! Your voice is an integral part of your sexuality and your pleasure. Opening your throat and making noise helps keep your body open and relaxed. It keeps you breathing. If you are concerned about roommates or neighbors listening in, soundproof your room as best you can. Play music. A towel at the base of the door can help to absorb sound. Masturbating in the shower can give you the privacy to use your voice freely.

4. Touch Your Whole Body

We often think of masturbation as simply getting off; and it can get very genitally focused. Attend to your whole body when you touch yourself. What kind of touch do you like on your legs or stomach? Do you like to touch your hair and face? Sexual energy moves throughout your entire body, not just your genitals. Explore its reaches.

Especially touch yourself in the places that feel the best *and* the places where you don't want to go. Usually the places we want to ignore hold valuable healing and information. Touch your face, your feet, your calves, your back, your belly, your vulva, your breasts, your anus, your butt, inside your vagina, your G-spot, your cervix, your thighs, the backs of your thighs. Come to know your body as you would want your greatest love to know your body.

I got comfortable touching my vulva first, then my arms and stomach. My breasts took a lot longer; I got really sad there. I slowly kept adding one more piece of my body back into the equation.—Angela

5. Stay Present and Embodied

Being present while masturbating translates into being present with a sexual partner. Many survivors talk about being dissociated during sex, floating away and out of their bodies and feelings.

Use the tools in chapter 3 on dissociation while you masturbate. While masturbating, focus on the sensations in your body. Notice warmth, coolness, relaxation, tension, tingling, surges of energy, numbness, areas of your body that are pulsating, and other areas that feel blank or void. What are you feeling in your feet? How about your lower back?

You can also practice being present by saying out loud what you are feeling and thinking: "I am moving my arms, it feels good to me to move my hips, I am feeling ashamed, I am worrying that my dead grandma can see me, I feel wetness in my vagina and this is exciting to me, this is scary to me, I am afraid I am not supposed to be doing this…" You can practice being present with yourself by being present with your experience.

When you notice yourself floating away, making grocery lists, bring yourself back. Breathe, notice the sensations in your body and the room you are in. Remind yourself why you are masturbating and what you want to get out of it.

Explore these Five Steps to Great Masturbation. For contrast, try masturbating while you stay very still and breathe shallowly. Make noise and then stop. Notice the difference.

How to Touch Yourself

You can try stroking, tickling, firm grabbing, and squeezing. As you become aroused, you'll find your body can take more intensity and firm touch. Experiment.

Here are some ideas for self-pleasuring:

- Massage yourself with warmed oil—don't forget your head and your feet!
- Alternate light and firm strokes down the length of your body.
- Lightly pull on your pubic hair or press on your pubic bone.
- Brush a feather or soft fabric over your body.
- Squeeze your nipples between your fingers or press your breasts into your chest with the palms of your hand.
- Firmly grab your areola, pull, play, and twist. Lick your fingers and wet your nipples and breasts.
- Touch your vulva by resting your whole hand over your genitals, and play with pressure.
- Feel your perineum, the soft skin between your vagina and anus.
- Massage your outer labia between your thumb and forefingers. Do the same with your inner labia.
- Pull your clitoral hood back to feel your clit. Rub your clit in small circles or up and down where it is most sensitive. See if you like rubbing it with the flat of your fingers, the tips, or your thumb.
- Get into the shower or bath and use the water pressure to stimulate your clitoris.

- Press your fingers or a dildo into your vagina. What are the different tex-tures? How do the different depths of your vagina feel?
- Stimulate your G-spot by pressing firmly into it with your fingers or a firm, slightly curved sex toy.
- Try a vibrator on your vulva, your clit, or your anus, or in your vagina.
- Masturbate by rubbing on the bed, a pillow, or a chair, or squeezing your legs together.
- Touch your anus on the outside. Explore the nerves there. Using water-based lubricant, explore the inside of your anus with your finger or a toy designed for anal play.
- Try nipple clips, dildos, a butt plug, or anal beads.
- Rub your arms and hands.
- Wrap your arms around yourself and hug yourself.
- Kiss your arms and knees.

A Masturbation Date

Set aside a regular time to be with yourself and masturbate. I suggest making a bimonthly date with yourself to discover and explore pleasure in your sexuality and your healing.

A self-pleasuring date might go like this:

Fix yourself your favorite dinner—just make sure you pick something that won't put you to sleep! Or you might gather fruits, breads, and cheeses to nibble on while you play.

Create a beautiful ambiance, as you would for a lover. Put on music, get your-self some flowers, light candles. Make sure the room is warm enough. Get out sex toys (if you have them), water-based lubricant, or any erotica you may enjoy.

Remind yourself why you choose to masturbate. Maybe tonight your inten-tion is to give yourself a lot of pleasure or to try a new toy. Another night your focus might be on healing a specific trigger.

Begin by stroking your whole body and breathing. Use your hands, velvet, a feather. Rub your head, feet, and calves. Touch yourself lightly and then more firmly. Spread lotion or a scented oil on your body.

Read an erotic story or poem you like. Watch your favorite erotic DVD.

Rock your hips, feeling the sensations spread throughout your body. Press your back into the bed or couch. Move around. Feel your whole body come alive.

Now touch your vulva. Press your hand against your clit. Tug on your pubic hair, and press your finger into your perineum. Touch your labia with one hand while the other strokes your stomach.

Rub your arms. Breathe deeply, letting the pleasure and relaxation in your body grow.

Tell yourself that you deserve this pleasure. Grant yourself permission. Remember that you are loved and loving yourself. Tell yourself how sexy you are!

Get out your vibrator and dildo. Wet the dildo with water-based lubricant and rub the tip of it around your vulva. Put the vibrator near the opening of your vagina and move slowly up toward your clit...

Now *you* make up the rest...

When you are ready to stop, *stop*.

Even if you got triggered, didn't come, felt silly, or didn't like that new sixty-dollar sex toy, give yourself some credit. You did it! Notice that you are well and that no harm came to you. Show yourself some appreciation!

Of course there are as many ways to masturbate as there are women. Your masturbation date may be more sensually focused, with no genital touching at all. Or you may orchestrate an elaborate S/M scene for one, with intense sensation play, numerous accoutrements, and imaginative fantasies. It's up to you. Do what supports *your* sexual healing.

Sex Toys, Fantasies, and Porn

Using sex toys, reading erotica, and watching pornography are all popular masturbation options. Many people fantasize when masturbating. Some folks fantasize about people they know, others about strangers or acquaintances.

How I masturbate has really changed over time. I used to not masturbate. Then I fantasized a lot about strangers or movie stars. I still like to do that, and I also like now to float in the sensations of all of it. I fantasize about my girlfriend now, too.—Jane

Be aware of how you are using fantasy and erotica. Are you enhancing your experience, bringing yourself into your body? Do your fantasies take you out of you body? Are they a way to escape yourself? You don't have to stop fantasizing to change how fantasy works for you. See chapter 12 for more information on fantasizing.

Fantasy has always been big in my life. It gets me out of my distracting thoughts and past the road blocks to my sexual response.—Terri

Compulsive Masturbation

Some survivors compulsively masturbate to fill needs that aren't necessarily sexual. You may masturbate to calm down or to deal with intense emotion. You may masturbate when you feel angry or afraid, or when you feel uncomfortably close to someone. Compulsively masturbating can be a way to try to temper or shut down emotions related to the abuse.

Sometimes incessant masturbating is a natural stage of healing. If you are masturbating more than you are comfortable with, check in with yourself. If you could have anything at all right now, what would it be? Do you want to masturbate? Do you want to be held? Are you hungry? Are you scared? If you want to masturbate, go ahead. If you need something else, give yourself that.

I masturbated incessantly during one part of my healing. I masturbated to memories and images of the abuse. Then when I was ready, it shifted. I didn't feel manic about it anymore and the abuse fantasies had lost their attraction. —Rosa

Mutual Masturbation

Mutual masturbation is masturbating with another person. One of you can masturbate while the other watches, or you can both masturbate together. There are
numerous benefits to mutual masturbation. It is one of the best ways to show your
partner how you liked to be touched. Some things are easier to show than to tell.
You can find out what turns your partner on. Mutual masturbation can also let
you play at being a voyeur or an exhibitionist, and it is the most foolproof form
of safer sex.

For many, the thought of masturbating with someone else is inconceivable.
Even in long-term marriages and partnerships, many people don't know how or
how often their partners masturbate.

*I think of masturbation as private. I would be embarrassed to reveal that much
of myself.—Evelyn*

*For me it feels safer to masturbate with a new lover before we are sexual with
each other. In the past I have been sexual with anyone who showed any interest whether I wanted to or not. This approach forces me to communicate with
a lover first, to get to know him better, and then to see if I want to really be
sexual with him.—Marty*

Mutual masturbation is a wonderful option when one of you does not want
to have partner sex but you both still want to be sexually intimate.

*My girlfriend and I are both incest survivors. We have not always been on the
same timeline when it came to our recovery and sex. One thing we came up
with when one of us did not want to have sex for a while was to hold the other
one while she masturbated. This became a way for us to keep sex in our relationship during harder parts of the healing.—JR*

Many people, survivors included, find watching or being watched a big turn-
on. It can be very exciting to watch your partner pleasure himself or herself in
front of you, or to get your partner all turned on by watching you.

I love getting my lover all hot just by watching me masturbate. I don't let him touch me until I say he can, no matter how steamy he gets. It is a great game.—Aurora

Sex Guide Exercises

1. Explore your beliefs about masturbation. What did you learn about masturbation? Who or what taught you that? If you could decide what masturbation is for you, what would you say?
2. Make a list of the top ten reasons to masturbate. How could it serve you and your sexual healing?
3. Create a Masturbation Discovery Log. Write down what you find you like and don't like. What works for you? What comes up as you masturbate? How do you feel in your body? How are you using masturbation to heal?

chapter seven

Consent and Boundaries:

The "Yes," "No," and "Maybe" of Sex

Boundaries are confusing. I am not really sure when to say "yes" and when to say "no." I mostly just follow the other person's lead in sex. Maybe they know what they want.—Jackie

I painstakingly came to realize that respecting my own boundaries around sex, saying "no" when I didn't want to have sex, and initiating sex when I did want it, was the fastest way for me to heal sexually.—Rebecca

What Is Consent?

Consent is the ability to choose, based on your own internal experience, what you want physically, emotionally, mentally, spiritually, and sexually, and then to communicate those wants. Consent is an ongoing process of making choices. This is what therapists mean when they talk about being "at choice." You can consent to one thing and not to another, or change your mind at any point in a sexual encounter. Between "yes" and "no," there is a huge territory, which I call the land of "maybe." "Maybe" is where you will do most of your work with boundaries.

To practice consent, you need to be in touch with the bodily sensations that let you know what you do and do not want. You need to know what you like sexually. You need enough information to make a decision that serves your interests. Finally, you need to know how to communicate your consent to your partners.

You can be hot and heavy into kissing, decide you are done for now, and choose to stop. You can be in the middle of oral sex and decide that you do not want to continue. You can say "maybe" to penetration, and later decide you do want to try it. You can say "yes" to sex as often as you like. You can ask for your stomach to be touched and your hips not. What you said "no" to last time might be a "yes" this time, and vice versa. This is a radical concept to most people, especially to survivors of childhood sexual abuse.

> I had no idea that I could say "no" to sex. I thought that once I started kissing someone, that was it; I had to do whatever they wanted or else I'd be a tease. I had a lot of sex I didn't want to have.—Marty

> I used to worry that changing my mind during a sexual experience would be too hard on my girlfriend. I started to practice saying what I wanted and didn't want as we went. She actually really liked it! Sometimes it slowed things down, but mostly it let us explore so much more. Our sex is a lot more interesting and hot now, and I feel known.—Kate

Having full say about your own body does not mean disregarding others' feelings. It means that you have full say over *you*, while others have the same say over *their* bodies and sexuality. Some survivors are so unaccustomed to having control over their own sexuality that they confuse choice with selfishness. "What about what the other person wants?" they ask. The other person's wants are just as valid and valuable as yours—just not *more* so. Find sexual experiences that will delight both of you, or don't be sexual together at all.

Sexual Abuse and Unwanted Sex

Nearly all the survivors I have worked with report having had sex when they didn't want to. It's almost as if this were taken for granted; unwanted sex becomes such a given for survivors that many hardly notice it anymore.

Childhood sexual abuse teaches you to disregard your own internal sense of boundaries and to run your life by somebody else's rules. When you were abused, you did not get the opportunity to act on your internal sense of consent. You were not invited to state your boundaries, and if you managed to express your feelings, you were not heard or respected.

Sexual abuse can also have the effect of turning consent upside down and inside out. "No" meant "yes," and "yes" meant "no." Saying "no" had no effect or may have brought on worse abuse. You may have been manipulated into asking for sexual contact. Sexual contact may have been your only source of comfort or connection.

"No" was clearly not an acceptable response to my father. The last time I tried to say "no" I was nine. I said "no" and my body froze, wouldn't cooperate. He became so outraged that he beat me, kicking me in the back, breaking my rib. "No" was no longer a possibility for me after this.—Laura

When I was seven, I asked my grandpa to play our "game" that he had taught me. It was a touching game. Before then he would tickle my back and I his, but this time he began touching my legs and my chest. He molested me. I always thought it was my fault.—Marianne

It is vital that you reintegrate the experience of choice and consent into your sex life. Regarding your body and soul, you are now the one who decides. You now have the first, middle, and last word on what you choose sexually.

I often hear people make exceptions to this. "You mean I can say 'no' to sex with my husband of eighteen years?" Yes, you can say "no" anytime you do not want to have sex. While you did not have a choice about unwanted sexual contact as a child, you now get to have full choice about the kind of sex you want to have, when you want to have it, where, and with whom.

Another survivor in a workshop realized, "These last years, as I have been coming into my sexuality, my partner has been judgmental about what I like sexually. He says something is wrong with me because my sexuality makes *him* uncomfortable. I am just fine. My desires are just fine. He doesn't have to do anything he doesn't want to, but I also don't have to limit myself based on his opinions."

People hold many unspoken rules about sex and consent: "You can't say 'no' too many times in a row before you have to say 'yes.' " "You can't initiate sex too often because people will think you're a nympho." "You have to finish what you started." Take a moment to reevaluate the rules you learned about consent both from the abuse and the culture at large. When are you *not* "allowed" to say "no"? When are you *not* "allowed" to say "yes" or initiate sex?

You never again have to have unwanted sex. You never again have to have sex based solely on another person's needs and desires—no matter how convincing your partner may be, no matter how much you may love your partner, not even if your partner threatens to leave you. From this moment on, *you* are the sole owner of your body and your sexuality.

Embodied Consent

The information that you receive from your body in the form of sensations, feelings, and intuition is key to the process of making choices. Survivors learn to

> ## Even if ...
>
> Even if...you have been married for twenty years, you can decline to have sex, whenever and as often as you like.
>
> Even if...you had sex with someone before, you can choose whether you want to have sex with him or her again.
>
> Even if...you have initiated sex twice already today, you can initiate sex again.
>
> Even if...you are turned on and have all your clothes off, you can choose to stop sexual activity.
>
> Even if...your partner does not want to try the things that you want, you can negotiate ways to express your sexuality on your own terms.
>
> Even if...your partner threatens to leave you, it is your choice not to be sexual.
>
> Even if...others think what you desire is strange, you can choose whatever sexual expression fits you.
>
> Even if...(add your own).

override their feelings and acquiesce to others' wishes. I want to invite you back into your body now. From inside your own body, you can decide what you want sexually based on your own needs, desires, and values. I call this embodied consent.

> *Consent was a good idea to me. It sounded right, but I didn't for the life of me know what that meant in the actual situation.*—Pam

The first step in embodied consent is noticing your own body sensations and signals. What are you feeling in your chest, your pelvis, your stomach? When you are doing something that you want to do, when your insides are saying "yes," how do you know this? For example, one survivor I worked with said her stomach relaxes and she gets a warm sensation there when she knows it is okay for her to go ahead. Another survivor reported that she felt an openness and warmth in her pelvis and a connection to her voice and throat when she felt a "yes." Check this out for yourself. How do you know when your body says "yes"?

Conversely, what signals and sensations appear in your body when you do not want to engage in a certain sexual experience? How do you know when it is not feeling right anymore? Another survivor reported: "I start to feel panicky in my chest and want to pull away physically. I usually try to talk myself into sexual contact, telling myself, 'what's the big deal? Nothing bad is happening.' Then if I don't listen to my body, I usually check out and have sex without being there." When you do not want to be sexual in some way, you may notice your breathing getting short, your stomach getting tight, or your body wanting to pull away. Pay attention. This is *you* communicating to you. What sensations in your body communicate a "no" to you?

And what about maybe? Sometimes there are a number of seemingly contradictory feelings happening in your body at once. You may feel sexually turned on in your hips and vulva, and feel pulled away in your chest. You may feel a warmth in your solar plexus, indicating the go-ahead, and be afraid or tight in your throat. What do you do then?

Actually, experiencing contradictory feelings is familiar territory for most survivors. Consent then becomes a matter of distinguishing what sensations are what. One workshop participant noted, "I feel the consent to be sexual in my belly, it is a settled, sure sensation, and I can feel anxious in my chest at the same time. I am anxious when I am getting close to someone. I can count on this happening. It does not mean I do not want to be sexual. It just means I am feeling scared while I am being sexual." Another survivor shared, "I usually stop having sex when my stomach gets tight. I see now, though, that my stomach being tight is me feeling stressed about being turned on. It was so awful to get turned on

during the sexual molestation that my body still tries not to do it. If I just relax
and acknowledge my stomach and the fear there, I can go right on being sexual.
My stomach being tight does not mean I do not want to have sex."

Sometimes we make choices about sex in our heads, because it seems like a
good idea, seems to make sense, when we may be feeling something entirely different in our bodies.

> I have sex when it seems right, like all the pieces are in place... I never even
> thought to check in with my body to see if I wanted to have sex.—Barb

> I didn't know I had a body, so I made almost all my decisions out of my head.
> I ignored my body just like I did when I was getting abused. It seemed like a
> morass of emotions and feelings that I didn't want anything to do with.—Rose

You can end up feeling used, angry, or self-loathing after such a decision.

Consent does not always *feel* comfortable, easy, and joyous. Sometimes a consensual sexual experience can bring up sadness, anger, or feelings of abandonment. It is important to learn the difference between experiencing feelings and
wanting to stop what you are doing. You can do this by paying attention to your
body and learning its language.

Informed Consent

To practice consent, you need outside information, too—*all* of the information
necessary to make a decision. You may need to know that your partner is willing to practice safer sex or that he or she is available for the type of relationship you desire. You may need to know that your partner will stay with you
through the messier moments of your healing process. What are *your* criteria for
having sex?

> I have finally learned to ask guys I am interested in if they practice safer sex
> before I have sex with them. What a concept!—Jackie

Here are some questions to ask your partner:

- Are you willing to practice safer sex? Have you been tested for sexually transmitted diseases? When? What were the results?
- I am interested in being nonmonogamous (or monogamous). Where do you stand on that?
- I am looking for a long-term relationship (or a summer fling). What are you looking for?
- What do you like sexually? I like oral sex (or lots of cuddling or anal penetration). Is this something you are interested in?

While these questions may seem rather forward, you can save yourself and others heartaches and headaches by learning to communicate about sex. You can have this conversation before you are sexual with a partner, early on in a sexual relationship, or after years in a marriage or long-term relationship.

The idea of actually talking about sex was a shocker. You mean, say all of this out loud? Luckily, I trusted the friend who kept encouraging this. I explored what I might want to say and realized that certain things were important to me about sex and that they were worth saying.—Evelyn

Knowing What You Want

Of course, you have to know what you want before you can tell someone else. Your desires are not an unchanging menu of sex acts. Rather, knowing what you want means knowing what feels pleasurable or hot to you, what you are interested in exploring, and what is scary yet intriguing to you.

As you articulate your desires, you can count on making mistakes. You will end up saying "no" to something you wish you had tried, and you will most likely say "yes" to something that you later discover you did not want.

When I first let myself start having sex, I didn't know where my boundaries were. When I messed up and had sex I didn't want to have, I felt awful—like now I was betraying myself. I kept trying, though, and was easier on myself

after a while. How was I supposed to be good at having boundaries when I was
never allowed to have one? I had to learn.—Naomi

Be your own strongest advocate and be gentle with yourself. Respect your
own sense of consent and boundaries as you would want the person you love most
to be respected. Give yourself room to explore and make mistakes.

Communicating Consent

My new mantra about sex is this: If you want it, say so; if you don't want it,
say so. It is up to me now to take care of me.—Rebecca

You may find it frightening to talk about sex—*especially* with the person you
want to have sex with. Yet good sexual communication is the single most important tool you can acquire to improve and empower your sex life. Communication
is *how* you consent

Take a moment now and practice saying aloud, "I would like to have sex with
you." Change the words if you want to, but imagine you are inviting someone to
have sex with you. Now try, "I might be interested in having sex with you; I'll get
back to you." And now, "I do not want to have sex with you." Change "have sex"
to another sexual activity and repeat the three statements: "I would like to kiss
you." "I might be interested in touching you." "I do not want to have intercourse
with you."

Now say these in front of a mirror. There you are, a person learning to talk
about sex! Talking about sex will become comfortable over time. At Good
Vibrations, I lost count of the number of times people thanked me for being able
to speak about sex as a normal and natural part of life. People were relieved to
hear me say "vulva," "clitoris," "penis," "anus," and "balls" without laughing or
having my voice crack. This normalization of sex and sexual terms came with
practice. Believe me, I wanted to giggle a lot during my training!

Once I learned that I deserve to be sexual when I want to and not when I don't,
then I had to learn how to say it. That was weird, and harder than I'd thought.

I would get all embarrassed and shy, and not want to speak. I had to do it anyway because I was not going to go ahead when I didn't want to anymore; I was tired of not asking for what I wanted.—Jo

Surprisingly, saying what I wanted sexually made me more nervous than saying "no." I thought, "Who am I to actually ask for the sex I want?" I did not feel deserving of it. I felt like a slut sometimes, and I felt shame that I was being so forward. This was all muck from the abuse that I had to work through. —Sheila

"Yes," "No," and "Maybe" Vignettes

The following are stories about consent that I have collected over time in my work with survivors and sexual healing. I include them here as examples of embodied consent and communication:

The "Yes"

I was becoming more comfortable with my sexuality and had been learning to masturbate. I had the idea that I'd like to invite my husband to watch me masturbate. So, I asked him. He was surprised and delighted. I watched him watching me, and I felt connected to him. It was much more exciting than I'd expected. I asked him to kiss me but not touch me while I continued to masturbate. I came that way, kissing him. It was a little scary and so good for me.

The "Maybe"

My girlfriend moved to another state to attend college and I stayed home because of work. We could only afford to see each other periodically, and things got pretty lonely. She suggested that we try phone sex, that we both get vibrators or dildos and masturbate with each other while talking

sexy over the phone. I was so uncomfortable when she asked. Instead of
saying "no," though, I said, "Maybe, give me a few days to think about
it." I thought about what made me so uncomfortable. I was scared that I
might sound silly, or that I might not be very good at it. Those weren't
good enough reasons for me to not do it, and I thought I could see it as
a new challenge. I was awkward at first, but it was so fun over time. I
learned so much about both of us sexually, and I became a lot more confident about sex and talking about sex by talking on the phone.

The "No"

A long-term co-worker asked me to dinner and propositioned me. He
actually put quite a lot of pressure on me to have sex. I clearly stated that
I wasn't interested. It took three times before he got it.

I was playing around with my lover. We'd only been lovers for a few
months and I hadn't talked about the incest much. He began to put his
mouth on my breast in a way that really reminded me of the abuse. I
didn't know what to do at first; then I took a deep breath and told him
that I really liked him touching me, but I didn't enjoy him sucking on my
breast like that. I told him I liked it better when he nibbled. It had taken
me a lot of sexual healing to get to the place where I could do that. I was
so proud of myself, and he did fine with it.

Negotiate Before You Play

In the S/M community, there is a practice of negotiating before any S/M or sexual play. The idea is to talk about your interests, your boundaries, your desires,
and safer sex before getting into the action. This practice can be empowering for
people of any sexual persuasion. Talking about sex before you do it gives you the
opportunity to create a sexual experience that includes your needs, desires, and
boundaries.

Whether you are engaging with a new sexual partner or someone you have been with for years, have a conversation about sex before you play. Choose a relaxed environment, not the bedroom or your usual sexual setting. The kitchen table can be a good spot. Or, take a drive or a walk. Talk with your partner about what you want, what you do not want, and where you feel there is room for exploring. Now is the time to talk about your criteria for safer sex. You can also use this time to bring up something you might like to change about your sex together. Ask the questions that are important to you, and find out about your partner's needs, limits, and desires. Together you can negotiate sex that will be satisfying for both of you.

> I was embarrassed to talk about my boundaries and ask questions before I was sexual. I felt like it would put a damper on the spontaneity of our attraction. It ended up being more of a turn-on, though, and I felt so much more comfortable talking during sex, too.—Tracy

Depending upon your level of intimacy with your partner, you can also choose to talk about how to handle any triggers that may come up during sex. You can tell her or him what you are like when you dissociate and what kind of support would be helpful. Chapter 11 discusses developing a trigger plan for sex that you can use as a template for this conversation.

Long-term partners may think that they know each other well enough to skip these conversations. I have found, however, that this is not usually the case. Partners can learn an amazing amount of new information about each other. If you are in a long-term marriage or partnership, what have you not told your partner about sex? How would you like to change or develop your sex life? What could you discover about your partner?

Response from Others

Whether or not your sexual partner is happy with your sexual boundaries or agrees with your sexual choices, you get to have them. Your needs and desires do not require someone else's permission. For many survivors, this is a difficult concept.

It's automatic for me. If I have a boundary that my lover doesn't like, I start figuring out how to change it, how to fit me to what he wants.—Janet

As a survivor, you may be unfamiliar with having your sexual boundaries noticed, let alone respected. One workshop participant said, "I think I fight more than I need to about sex. I assume that my boyfriend wants me to do things I don't want to do. When I check it out with him, that's not really true."

Whatever the response, you are free to make your own decisions and take the action necessary to back them up. As an adult, you can act on your own behalf in ways that you could not as a child when you were powerless to stop the abuse.

If your sexual partner does not respect your boundaries, you can take action to protect yourself. You have a number of options.

You can restate your boundary and a consequence for it not being respected: "I want to use a condom when we have sex. If you are unwilling to do that, I won't have sex with you."

You can leave the sexual situation in order to talk in a nonsexual setting: "I want to talk to you about this more, but outside of bed. I'm going to put my clothes on and I'll meet you in the kitchen."

You can leave the situation altogether: "This is not okay for me. I am leaving now."

If your partner is uncomfortable with your sexual choices, she or he may try to make you feel bad about your desires. You do not have to collapse into your partner's opinion or mold yourself to fit his or her values. Again, you have options.

You can ask your partner to read sex education books or watch educational DVDs to learn more about the type of sex you are interested in.

You can invite your partner to explore new territory together.

You can also choose to change the nature of your relationship and engage sexually with someone else who shares your sexual interests. You get to create the sex life that works for you!

When you chose sexual partners, pay attention to their willingness to support your boundaries. Are they able to encourage your sexual desires even if your desires are different from their own? Remember, actions speak louder than words.

Do you respect your own boundaries and sexual desires? Do you edit your needs or think of yourself as bad for having your desires? Practice respecting yourself as you ask others to respect you.

Healthy Risks

Healthy risks are choices that take into account both your well-being and your desire for growth. Pushing up against old limitations in order to allow more pleasure and choice into your sex life is key to sexual healing. Healthy risks push you past your comfort zone without challenging you beyond what you can handle.

> *Sexual healing is a step-by-step process for me. I push through a barrier, usually feeling terrified, get to a new plateau, then push through another barrier. It reminds me of the tortoise and the hare; slow but steady wins the race.* —Laurie

Many survivors say that they just want sex to feel safe. Unfortunately, having as your goal sex that is unthreatening and comfortable will keep you stuck. Because of the nature of sexual abuse and trauma, as you heal sexually, you will necessarily pass through times of discomfort and fear. As you take healthy risks that increase your pleasure and your choices, you will feel all the old fear, loss, and anger. This is normal. With each new sensation you allow yourself to feel, your sexuality will be freed from the control of sexual abuse.

> *I think healing means feeling good. I start to feel bad and I think I must be back-sliding. My group tells me it is the opposite—that I will feel worse at times when I am getting better. It's like cleaning out a wound.* —Marianne

What is your default behavior? Do you automatically say "no" to sex? Or do you say "yes" without asking yourself whether you even want it?

If you are more likely to say "no" to sex or new sexual experiences, taking a healthy risk may mean pushing the envelope. What is one risk you can take sexually that will bring more freedom and choice into your sex life? You may want to risk buying some sexy clothes, and even wearing them on a date. Maybe you can risk initiating a sexual experience of your own design, or even a conversation with your lover about sex. What will expand the constraints on your sexual expression, while not pushing you beyond what you can handle?

If you are more likely to say "yes" and have a harder time finding "no," a healthy risk for you may be setting a sexual boundary. You might risk not having sex if you don't want to—when you might have otherwise talked yourself into it. You might say "no" to a new sexual experience that would push you too far. Maybe you could have a conversation with your lover about your boundaries. What would you say "no" to if you could say "no" to anything without any negative consequences?

Sex Guide Exercises

1. Consider two consensual sexual experiences you've had. What sensations and signals in your body, emotions, and thought process let you know they were consensual?

2. Consider two nonconsensual sexual experiences. What sensations and signals in your body, emotions, and thought process let you know they were nonconsensual? Did you dissociate? When and how?

3. Practice saying your "yes," "no," and "maybe" about sex out loud: "I would like to _____." "I might like to _____. I do not know if I want to _____." "No, I do not want to _____." Fill in the blanks with your own sexual desires and boundaries. Start by saying these out loud to yourself, then try practicing with a friend. It gets easier quickly with a little practice.

4. Consider two healthy sexual risks. How will these risks serve your sexual healing? Who can support you in taking these risks? How can you take care of yourself in the process?

5. What forms of safer sex do you use? What is your risk level for contracting a sexually transmitted disease? What are your standards for safer sex in your sexual relationships?

chapter eight

Partner Sex

Sex with my lover can be the most pleasurable or the most terrifying experience.—Aurora

Sex with a partner can be a way to connect deeply with another human being, to get off, or to be silly or playful. Sex can even be a way to heal. The purpose of sex is not necessarily penetration or orgasm; you can have great sex without either one. Nor is sex limited to vaginal penetration of a woman by a man—fine as that might be. Sex can involve kissing, touching, oral sex, anal sex, holding, S/M—or any of the above. Sex is really what you want it to be. Sex is now up to you, your desires, and your creativity.

Like masturbation, good partner sex takes practice and learning. Most of us get very little quality information about sex, yet we assume we are supposed to know magically how to do it. With quality information and a willingness to experiment, you can create the sex life you desire.

I learned so much being exposed to the sex-positive community. Suddenly I knew all this neat stuff about sex. Now I have words to use, and ideas to try out.—Terri

Of course, partner sex can bring up old feelings, sensations, and triggers about your past sexual abuse. While this can be painful and frustrating, it can also be one of the most wonderful opportunities for healing.

My sex life has expanded by doing this healing work. I used to think sex was about intercourse and then it was over. I like things that I never knew I would, like giving head and anal sex. Now I am learning about tantra, and I've even tried phone sex.—Naomi

The Good, the Bad, and...the Pleasurable?

I have found that most survivors of childhood sexual abuse, no matter what their sexual preference or orientation, feel that what they do sexually is somehow wrong, deficient, perverted, or just plain *bad.* Sound familiar? Survivors I have worked with are concerned that the abuse has made them too sexually expressive, not sexually expressive enough, too conventional, or gay!

There are many connections between childhood sexual abuse and your sexual choices and problems. Perhaps most problematic is this belief that no matter what you want or don't want, you are bad. This feeling of being bad is a result of the abuse, which caused you to internalize shame and self-blame. Many survivors do not give themselves permission to explore sexually for this reason. Contrary to your beliefs, your sexuality is not bad and you did nothing wrong.

Each time I would go out on a limb and enjoy myself sexually, I would feel like I had been too wild, or too expressive, and I would try to tone it down. I am really very conventional about sex, so I don't know what I felt was so wrong, besides the sheer fact of enjoying it.—Evelyn

I express myself sexually in lots of ways that are unconventional. I am into S/M and I am bisexual. I have felt bad about this, like I am fucked up, or wrong. I have worked on just accepting me—accepting that what turns me on turns me on and I like what I like.—Janie

I blather on about how much I want joy and sex in my life; then when I get it, I turn around and run screaming in the other direction.—Maria

Your Sex Basics Checklist

So how do you determine when sex is good for you? When it's okay to follow your desires? Or even whom to have sex with? There are basic principles you can follow that can help you establish a healthy basis for your sexuality. You can use the following checklist to help you consider the sex you are having, or are interested in having, or to help steer yourself through confusing turns or triggers in a sexual encounter.

1. Breathe.

Are you breathing? Is your breath shallow or filling your belly and chest? Breathe while you are talking about sex or even thinking about sex. This way, you'll get into the habit of being relaxed and present when being sexual.

2. Stay in Your Body.

Can you feel sensations in your chest, arms, and legs? Move around if you need to. Feeling your body becomes your reference point for knowing what you want and where your boundaries are.

3. Be Present.

Are you in the room? Notice your surroundings. Are you present with yourself? What is your mood, what are your thoughts? Remind yourself, *Here I am, I am here*. Are you present with your partner? Notice your partner. Look at her or him. Your partner is there with you.

4. Practice Consensual Sex.

Is this sex consensual for all parties? Do you want to be doing what you are doing? Remember, you can be afraid and still want to engage in sex. And you can feel aroused physically even when you are doing something you don't want to be doing. Ask yourself if your decision to be sexual is based upon your own needs and desires. That is the place to say "yes" from. Remember that "yes," "no," and "maybe" are all valid responses to any given sexual situation.

5. ENSURE YOUR SAFETY.

Check your physical, mental, and emotional safety. Are you sober and drug-free? Is your partner? Are you in a place that is safe for you? You may feel afraid if you are triggered or if you are taking a risk sexually, but this is different from being unsafe. Do you have the power in the current situation to take care of yourself, to ensure your own well-being physically, emotionally, and sexually? If the answer is "yes," then you are most likely in a safe situation.

6. PRACTICE SAFER SEX.

Have you assessed your risk for sexually transmitted diseases with your partner? Are you acting on this information, using safer-sex measures? If your partner refuses to practice safer sex, he or she does not get to have the wonderful opportunity to be sexual with you. Period.

As you can see, this checklist is not about whether it's okay to like bondage, or kissing, or having sex with more than one person at a time. You can decide what is acceptable and enjoyable for you. Who else would know that? What this checklist will do is help you build an embodied, self-referential sexuality, one in which you are in your body, present for the experience, and doing what you love, enjoy, like, and want, based upon your own needs. What a concept, huh?

Mistakes

Using this approach will mean exploring. You may be in your body and breathing during sex for the first time. This can be a strange and unfamiliar experience. You will probably make mistakes along the way, even do things you realize later that you didn't want to do. As when learning anything new, you'll get better at partner sex with practice. Your mistakes are an essential part of the learning process.

I had sex with a woman when I didn't want to. She sucked on my breasts in a way that really triggered me, and I didn't tell her to stop. I took the "bear it till it's over" approach. I felt horrible for days. I felt like I had betrayed myself, my little girl, in a way I'd promised I never would. I finally dealt with it by apolo-

gizing to myself and holding my breasts tenderly, washing the experience out of them. I realized I am learning. Although I have been so sexualized, I have had little sex that was about and for me.—Kathy

Choosing Sexual Partners

You can choose your partners based upon your desires, needs, and values. Can your prospective partner give you what you are looking for in a sexual partnership? Do you want a fling, someone to date, a lover, or a life partner? Do you care if your partner is sexual with others? Do you want to be sexual with others as well? Do you want an emotionally intimate relationship? Does this person have the capacity for that? Does this person like tantra, S/M, lunchtime quickies, tender evenings of lovemaking, or any other form of sexual expression you may prefer? Do you want to invite your partner to be involved in your sexual healing? Will you tell him or her about your abuse? These are questions to ask yourself and to talk about with your partner.

I never thought much about what I wanted from a lover. I'd just be attracted to someone, or more often, someone would ask me out and I'd go. I'd have sex with them until I realized I didn't necessarily like it—or until it would just end.—Marie

What do I want from a lover? This is a good question. I have been involved with a number of people with whom I wasn't sexually compatible. I am just now saying this is a priority for me.—Rain

When you enter into a new sexual relationship, notice whether your partner's behavior matches his or her words. Behavior is the proof in the pudding. What does this mean? It means knowing what you want and watching to see if the other person can offer it to you. This is not a test but rather a way of being awake to the potential (*and* limitations) of the relationship.

Talk about what you want, talk about what your partner wants, and watch your partner's and your own behavior. Your intentions for caring for each other may be fabulous, but your behavior will reveal what you each are able to give and receive right now.

Many survivors build relationships on hope and projection, settling for a fraction of what they want because at least it is something. When you are used to being mistreated, or unused to being loved and cared for, a little can look like a lot. Keep returning to your heart's desires. Don't be afraid to hope for your wildest dreams. Your dreams may not come true in exactly the form you expect, but they will serve as a guide to better choices. The more good things you expect for yourself, the more you can align your actions with your dreams, and the more likely you are to get what you want.

I have learned and learned well to find out what I want and go for it. It has been tricky to receive it once it comes, however. I get uncomfortable and start to doubt whether I deserve it or not. I want to pull away.—Anna

I always seem to fall in love with people who aren't available. One was married, another emotionally unavailable. I am not really attracted to people who are ready for a relationship, it seems.—Jo

Trust

Because childhood sexual abuse violates trust, trust can be a tricky topic for most survivors. Some survivors grant trust to people long before they have earned it, and others do not trust even those whose trustworthiness has been demonstrated. When you are looking to trust someone, consider these three factors: competency, consistency over time, and a congruency between words and behavior.

I thought trust was some objective thing that was "good" to do. So I just trusted everyone. This of course was a bad idea, because there are people out there who aren't trustworthy, or with whom I don't want to be that intimate.— Melanie

Ask yourself whether the person in question is competent or has the skills and tools you want. Look for competence in the areas that are important to you.

Someone may be competent at playing the piano but not competent at knowing how to communicate about sex and healing. Of course, your partner can learn new skills if she is committed to doing so, and this means that your trust in that area may build as she becomes better at it.

> ### Trust
>
> 1. Competency.
> 2. Consistency.
> 3. Congruence between words and deeds.

Trustworthiness is also shown when someone is consistent over time. If someone promises you that he will respect your boundaries and does so consistently over time, than he can earn your trust.

Last, trust is built when someone's words match her actions. Does she do what she says she will? If someone consistently says one thing and does another, there is not much room for building trust.

Let's Talk About Sex

You don't have to wait until you get into the bedroom to talk about sex. Please don't wait, in fact. If you do, you'll be missing out on the most important tool for creating the sex life you want—communication.

Learning to talk about sex will increase your satisfaction with your sex life more than any other technique. If you spend the next year just focused on learning how to talk about sex and sexual healing, you will have given your sex life a huge boost.

Communication involves some self-knowledge and willingness to share that with another. The more experienced you are with your own desires, the ways you like being touched, and your own process of recovery, triggers, and healing, the easier the communication and interaction with another will be.

> Knowing how to talk about sex has been the most empowering thing for me. I can tell my partners what I like and want; I can be responsible for my own pleasure by communicating.—Anna

> Negotiating scenes with my lovers is so amazing. I have complete say now as to what is going to happen, what will turn me on, and how to be with me if I

get triggered. I tell my lovers up front what the signs are if I am getting triggered and how far I can push my boundaries there.—Rebecca

When talking about sex with a partner or potential partner, some simple rules prove useful:

First, talk about sex outside of the place where you are going to have sex. Sit at the kitchen table, talk over a cup of coffee at a café, or take a walk. This will assist you both in becoming more comfortable integrating sexual talk into everyday settings, and you will not be quite as vulnerable as when you're naked, halfway into something hot and heavy. Before having sex is the time to talk about safer-sex practices as well.

Second, speak positively about sex, your desires, yourself, and your partner. We all tend to take feedback about sex very personally at first. If you want your partner to try something new or to change something he does, first let him know how much you like him touching you. Then add that you'd like to try something new or change the touch.

Third, be as specific as possible in your communication. This takes practice for most people. Use specific sexual words, such as *penis, ass, vulva, pussy, clit, breasts, nipples, anus, dick, G-spot, tongue, vagina,* and *prostate.* Practice saying these words aloud now. Go ahead, just say them. Add your own, too. Let yourself laugh. Most of us still feel silly learning how to talk about sex.

When talking about your desires, or fantasies, or asking your partner for a certain touch, be concrete and specific. For example, you might say that you like your clit touched in a circular motion on the left side, or that you do not like your clit stimulated directly but prefer the touch to be lower down, underneath it. If you like to be penetrated and then use a vibrator to take yourself over the top, spell that out. The more you communicate, the more satisfying your sexual experience will be and the more likely your partner will be to relax and join in.

I finally took a deep breath and told her, "I love it when you use your teeth on my nipple and when you roll my nipple between your fingers; that feels great. I don't like it when you suck my whole breast into your mouth. It feels uncom-

fortable to me." I thought she would freak out, but she didn't. She was glad to know what I liked and what I didn't.—Jeanie

As you let your sexual partner know what you like, showing her may also help. Getting around someone else's anatomy is not as easy as you might think. Show your partner how you like to be touched. Let her hand rest on yours to pick up the rhythm or the pressure.

It can be hard to explain how I like my clit touched. I like some pressure, but not too much, and I like it to the side of my clit, not directly on it. I have turned showing my lover how and where I want him to touch me into a sexy game. —Cheryl

In S/M, sex scenes are negotiated before the play begins. Sex partners talk about what they want, and maybe share fantasies or what they hope to heal. Whether you are into S/M or not, you can use this approach. Try planning out a sexual encounter with your partner before you begin. What are your sexual fantasies? What would make it a great experience?

Safer sex also takes communication. It is important to assess your risk level and plan what you are going to use for safer sex before you are sexual. You then have the chance to handle any disagreements and gather supplies before you are in the middle of sex. If you need to reassess or to demand that someone comply with safer sex smack dab in the midst of the action, please do so.

The Fear of Sex Talk

If talking to your sex partner about sex freaks you out, you are not alone. Most folks, survivors or not, are very uncertain about how to talk about sex. Communicating well about sex is a learned skill. A good way to get your feet wet is to read sex education books and erotica to see that people actually do talk openly about sex. This is also a great way to pick up vocabulary words and different styles for talking about sex. Then it's a matter of trying it yourself.

You can start by writing a list of sexual words you are uncomfortable with, and in the privacy of your own space, practice saying them aloud. Try out words you might not necessarily use, or words that you think are too risqué, like *cunt* or *cock*. Next, practice saying what you want: "I would really like you to touch my breasts and firmly squeeze my nipples," or "I'd like you to press your hips into me." It may seem terrifying at first, but you'll be amazed at how quickly you catch on. Communicating about sex allows you to get more of what pleases you and give your partner more of what pleases her or him. It is one of those win-win situations.

> *Sex got so much better when I learned to speak up. I used to try to silently adjust myself to make something feel better, which didn't always work. I read a couple of books about sex, and that helped a lot. I saw that other people can talk about it, so I figured I can, too.*—Maria

Disclosure: To Tell or Not to Tell

For many survivors, there is the question of whether or not to tell a sexual partner about your experience of abuse. If you are in a long-term intimate relationship, I encourage you to tell your partner. If you are uncomfortable doing so or you don't want to, I suggest you take a look at that fear and at your relationship. An intimate partnership can be a supportive and loving place to heal. And all of you gets to be loved and appreciated now, including the truth of your history. You no longer need to hide yourself away from those you are close to.

> *I am comfortable talking about the incest I experienced, but I take much longer and require more trust with a person before I am willing to talk about my experiences of ritual abuse. I waited a year into my relationship with my girlfriend to tell her about it.*—Rose

Because of the secrecy of childhood sexual abuse and the destruction of healthy boundaries, survivors tend to default to isolation or overexposure. Some survivors never tell anyone about what happened to them, tucking it away from present-day life. This keeps a survivor isolated and still in shame. Other survivors tell everyone about their abuse or disclose more information than a relationship is ready for. Many survivors who overexpose have a hard time keeping intimate friends and relationships.

When do you tell? A good time to tell is after you have established some trust with your partner. If you are entering a new partnership, and you want to know if your potential partner can handle being involved with a survivor who is healing, you may speak about your history sooner rather than later. Be prepared for any number of responses. Partners will have their own capacities for being able to hear about sexual abuse.

How to Meet Sexual Partners

The how and where of meeting sexual and intimate partners depends, of course, on what you are looking for. Do your homework by thinking about what is important to you in a sexual mate. The clearer you are about your criteria, the easier the process will be.

Most people meet their sexual partners at school or work, or through their friendship circles and communities. If you are serious about wanting a sex partner or mate, alert your friends and others in your social network. Tell them what you want and why. People love to play matchmaker.

Look for sexual partners in places where you do things you enjoy doing already. Where do you feel most yourself or most empowered? Start there. You might meet potential partners in business or personal development classes, clubs that interest you, your sports team, an outdoor club, online chat rooms, or a volunteer job. Some people place personal ads or use phone, online, or professional dating services.

If you are looking specifically for a sexual play partner, you may want to try phone sex lines, online discussion groups, sexual play parties, or a sex-focused club or political organization. While play parties and sex-focused organizations are usually located in larger cities, online discussion groups and phone sex lines are widely available.

Flirting and Kissing

Flirting and kissing are among the great pleasures of life. You can flirt with a glance or a brief conversation, or by sharing a momentary exchange of energy with someone who attracts you. Your kisses can be friendly and sensual or sizzling with eroticism.

I can kiss for hours. I like bringing all of my focus into my lips, and my lips touching hers. We play a game where we are not allowed to go beyond kissing for an entire date. The variety of kisses you can find when you are not in a rush to move on is amazing.—Pamela

Kissing and flirting, like any other aspect of sex, are learned skills. Can you remember your first consensual French kiss? Did you know what you were doing? Most of us didn't.

I French kissed a boy for the first time in sixth grade. I really wanted to. I was coming into my own desire. It was wet and sloppy; I didn't know to swallow my saliva. It was pretty messy, but also erotic.—Roslyn

You can discover many enjoyable ways to kiss. Try kissing with more or less pressure. Try changing how you use your tongue by making it softer or more firm. Explore by using your teeth and nibbling on your partner's lips. Ask your partner how he would like to be kissed. Try that. Let your partner know what about her kisses you like and how you would like to be kissed.

Finally speaking up for myself about kissing was a huge deal. I used to hate how my boyfriend kissed me, and I wouldn't say anything. It didn't feel intimate, but felt more like something I wanted to get away from. He was angry and ashamed when I finally told him that I didn't like our kissing. But we worked it through and tried different ways to kiss that made me feel like I wanted to be there.—Debbie

Go Out There and Have Fun!

Sex plays numerous roles in our lives. It is a way to be incredibly close with another, to relax and release, to get off and feel good, and to heal. As you heal sexually, remember to get out there and have some fun with sex, too. Whether you are engaging in sexual healing by yourself, with a partner, or with a number of lovers, sex can be fun, funny, silly, engaging, and expansive. Through learning about sex, you can begin to understand in your body that sex is no longer a weapon being used against you. Sex can be pleasurable and support your well-being.

Sex Guide Exercises

1. What do you want in a sexual partnership? Do you want to date? Do you want a long-term partnership? Do you want to introduce different ways of having sex into your current relationship? Let yourself brainstorm numerous possibilities. If you could have your heart's desire, what would that be? Write about this in your journal for at least fifteen minutes.

2. In a neutral, nonsexual setting, talk to your sexual partner or a friend about what you like or want to try sexually.

3. Set up a sex date with your sexual partner during which you agree not to have penetrative or oral sex. Use the time to explore other ways of touching and being together sexually.

4. As you are sexual with your partner or lover, attend to being present in your own body. Feel the sensations in your whole body, from your arms to your legs, head, and feet. Where do you notice sensations? Where are you blank or void? Where is it comfortable to feel? Where do you want to move away from your sensation? Can you be attentive to the sensations in your body and be with your partner at the same time?

5. Write in a journal about what you have noticed and learned. Keep practicing.

chapter nine

Oral Sex

Even though I was made to perform oral sex during my abuse, I love it now. It is one of my favorite ways to give to my partner.—Aurora

I still can't stand someone going down on me. This is how my stepfather would get me aroused, and I blank out when I try.—Barb

Oral sex is mouth-to-genital or mouth-to-anus sex. It involves kissing, sucking, licking, or nibbling your partner's penis, clitoris and vulva, or anus—or your partner licking yours. The official name for mouth-to-penis sex is *fellatio*; slang terms include *giving head, blow job,* and *sucking cock.* Cunnilingus is mouth-to-vulva-and-clitoris sex. *Going down on a woman* and *eating her out* are slang terms for cunnilingus. *Rimming* is slang for analingus, or mouth-to-anus sex.

Oral sex gets a bad rap socially. It is still on the books as illegal in some states, even between married couples in private. In sexual behavior surveys, however, the majority of people report that they practice oral sex. Many people rate oral sex as their favorite sexual activity.

Some people are concerned about cleanliness, or strong smells and tastes associated with oral sex. You can take care of this by washing thoroughly before oral sex or by using latex barriers.

There are lots of ways to learn about oral sex. Numerous books have come out in recent years that provide quality information and are good reads. How-to

DVDs are also available on the subject. Of course, the best way to learn about your partner's likes and dislikes regarding oral sex is to ask. Ask your partner to be specific about his or her likes. If your partner can't give you specifics, try different touches and ask for feedback.

Cunnilingus

Okay, girlfriends, cunnilingus it is. I remember that when I first learned about cunnilingus as a kid, I thought it sounded like one of the grossest things I could imagine. Funny, how things look a bit different from an adult perspective.

Cunnilingus can include licking, sucking, and nibbling on the clitoris, the labia, or the whole vulva. Many women like to be penetrated with fingers or a dildo while receiving oral sex. The tongue can also be used for penetration, but naturally it can go only so far.

There are many ways to go down on a woman. Different pressure, placement of the tongue, and rhythms are enjoyable for different women. Ask you partner what she likes best. Tell him what works for you. Do you like your entire vulva to be licked? Do you like the tongue to be flat, or do you enjoy the tip of the tongue? Do you like stimulation directly on your clitoris, to one side, or on the hood? Most women appreciate a steady rhythm and pressure just before and through orgasm. Changing tactics or pressure right before a woman comes usually doesn't work well.

Getting head (that's my name for getting eaten out) is the only way I can come with a partner.—Daren

Having my husband go down on me is both relaxing and such a turn-on. I love it!—Sally

Not everyone likes cunnilingus. Some feel that it is dirty "down there" and not a place where you want to put your mouth. This myth of the vulva being dirty still has a hold in our culture, although your mouth actually carries many more bacteria and germs than your vulva. Some people also find cunnilingus triggering because of past abuse, and others simply don't like it.

That is how my perp would make me have an orgasm. Then, of course, he would say I liked it and the whole thing was my fault. That is so fucked up. How was him manipulating me and my body my fault? I am still uncomfortable with someone going down on me, though. I lose track of where I am and who it is.—Liz

I like getting it, but I don't like giving it. This doesn't always go over well with my girlfriend.—Jeanie

Cunnilingus involves a certain kind of surrender. Your partner is focusing on you and your pleasure. As a survivor, this can be challenging for you to take in.

I used to worry about time when my fiancé was going down on me. I thought he must be bored, or that I was taking up too much time. I am slowly getting it that he is disappointed when I pull him away from doing that. He told me once that he could go down on me for an entire day. I was amazed.—Aurora

The How-to's of Cunnilingus

You may want to dive right in, but you'll most likely enjoy receiving or giving oral attention to the whole body. Experiment! As you become aroused, you'll be able to take more intense direct clitoral stimulation.

Whether you're receiving your lover's best oral attentions or going down on your girlfriend, the following are some places to begin. You can share these suggestions with your partner or try them out yourself:

- Kiss and stroke the nipples. Gently suck them until they become erect.
- Kiss and lick the belly, back, rear end, and inner thighs. Take your time; enjoy all that appreciation!
- Nibble at her armpits.
- Blow warm air gently across the vulva. (Never blow air directly into the vagina.)
- Caress the entire vulva with hands and face.
- Wrap her up with Saran wrap like a giant gift!

- Pull out a dental dam, put a little lube on your side of the latex, and hold it in place for your partner.
- Gently suck her clitoris.
- Open her outer vaginal lips with your fingers and lick up the center of the vulva from her vaginal opening to her pubic mound.
- Press your tongue flat against her clit. Move gently from side to side.
- Ask him to circle your clit with his tongue.
- Flick your tongue rapidly against the glans, hood, and shaft of her clitoris.
- Watch those teeth—ask her if she likes the feel of you nibbling on her inner thigh, labia, nipples, and even the hood of her clit.
- Press your tongue into her vagina.
- Give her clit a little snap: suck the dental dam into your mouth and then release it.

Cunnilingus and Triggers

If you like cunnilingus but it triggers you, or you don't like it now but would like to learn to, here are some practical suggestions. First, become familiar with your own genitals. Cunnilingus is a close-up on the vulva, after all. Use a mirror to look at yourself. What colors are your labia and clitoris? What is your hair like? Pull back your clitoral hood and check yourself out. Smell and taste your own vaginal secretions. You will notice that both the consistency and the taste of your fluids will change with your menstrual cycle. Your nutrition will also affect the taste of your secretions. Looking at yourself regularly is also a great way to track vaginal health. You will notice yeast and other infections by the changes in secretion and smell.

Next, introduce your partner to your genitals. Without letting him touch you, show your partner your vulva. Point out your clit and clitoral hood, your labia, and your vagina and perineum. Show her how and where you like to be touched by touching yourself. When you are ready, have your partner place his head near your vulva. Again, no touching yet. Remember to breathe. Practice staying in your body by feeling your sensations. Being in consistent eye contact and communication with your partner also helps. Talk about how this feels for you, and listen to your partner tell you his experience. This exercise can help you to build a new relationship to your own vulva, and to a partner's touch.

When you want to move into oral sex, find a position that feels powerful or comfortable for you. Many survivors find it useful to be in a position that allows eye contact. Your partner can kneel or lie between your legs, or you can kneel over his face. In the latter position, you can more easily control the contact and move a bit more freely. Try keeping your eyes open. This can help you orient in time and space and keep you present. Keep breathing. Stop when you want to stop, and continue when you are ready.

If you have never tried cunnilingus or do not want to try it, explore why not. What about it turns you off? What are your fears and concerns? Are there memories or traumas you associate with cunnilingus? Utilize the resources in chapter 11 on triggers to work more deeply on freeing cunnilingus for yourself. You may decide in the long run that you don't like cunnilingus—or you may find that you love it! What is most important is that you are making your own choice about it.

Fellatio

Many men enjoy receiving oral sex, and many women and men enjoy giving it. You will find that the head of the penis, or glans, and the coronal ridge surrounding it tend to be the most sensitive. The seam running down the underside of the penis, called the *raphe*, is the most sensitive part of the shaft. The shaft, otherwise, isn't very responsive to the tongue. Stroking the shaft of the penis with your hand, adding pressure or an up-and-down motion can be enjoyable for your partner. Sucking his balls is another favorite technique for many men. Most men agree that keeping the teeth out of the fellatio experience is best; they hurt!

I like giving my husband blow jobs. I like being able to take him like that; he melts.—Rona

If you use sex toys, you can give head to your partner's dildo. Strapping on a dildo and receiving an expert blow job is a fun erotic fantasy for many women, whatever the gender of their partner.

One of my greatest fantasies is imagining my girlfriend giving me a blow job.
Of course I don't have a penis, but when we fantasize about it out loud it sure
seems like I do.—JR

Some survivors like fellatio and others do not. Fellatio is often depicted as
a degrading act a woman is forced to perform. Many survivors *were* forced to
perform oral sex on their perpetrators, but while you may think that those who
were abused in this way would not like oral sex as adults, this isn't the case.
Many survivors who were abused orally as children are able to enjoy oral sex as
adults.

The How-to's of Fellatio

Take your time and discover the pleasures of your partner's body— for both his
enjoyment and yours. You can kiss, lick, suck, and caress. You can take your partner's penis as deeply into your mouth *as is comfortable for you.* You can pull his
penis out of your mouth before he ejaculates, if that is what you prefer. Here are
some ideas for exploring fellatio:

- Kiss and stroke his chest and nipples.
- Gently suck his nipples until they become erect.
- Lick his belly, back, butt, and inner thighs. Show him how much you
  appreciate him!
- Nibble at his armpits.
- Caress his balls and inner thighs with your hands and face.
- Pop an unlubed condom into your mouth and using your tongue and lips,
  roll it over the head of his penis. (You can practice on a dildo or zucchini.)
  Use your hands to roll it all the way down his shaft.
- Lick his penis from the base of the shaft to the glans and circle the head
  with your tongue.
- Suck firmly on just the head of the penis.
- Holding the base of the penis, relax your throat and bring your partner
  deeper into your mouth and throat. You can do this with a dildo, too.

- Press your tongue flat against his perineum (the area between his anus and balls).
- Nibble gently on the loose skin of his balls. You can suck on his balls and carefully take them into your mouth.

Fellatio and Triggers

If you like giving head but it triggers you, or if you don't like it now but would like to learn to, here are some suggestions: Become familiar with your partner's penis and balls. Take your time. Ask him to show you his genitals when his penis is not erect. Check out the colors and textures. Get to know his genitals in a way that lets you make friends with them. Begin to build a new association with male genitals. This is the body of someone whom you are choosing as an adult to be sexual with. Connect his genitals with him, and what you like, love, or care about in him. This penis is not here to hurt you. It is a part of his body through which you can both experience pleasure. Remember to breathe during this exploration, and practice staying in your body by feeling your sensations.

Don't plan on having oral sex initially. Use your hands to feel the various textures of his skin. Place your head close to him and become acquainted with his smells. You can kiss his genitals and taste them. Breathe. Remember that his genitals are a part of what you care about in him.

When you are ready to move into oral sex, find a position that feels powerful or comfortable for you. Many survivors find it useful to be in a position that allows eye contact. While he lies on his back, try kneeling next to him or between his legs. Keep your eyes open. This can help you orient in time and space and keep you present. Place your hand around the base of his penis; this way you can control the depth and speed of the movement. Keep breathing. Stop when you want to stop, and continue when you are ready. It is fine to remove your mouth before your partner comes, whether or not you are using condoms.

Utilize the resources in chapter 11 on triggers to work more deeply on freeing up fellatio for yourself. You may decide in the long run that you don't like fellatio—or you may find that you love it. What matters most is that you make your own choice about it. *You* choose your sex life now, not the abuse, not the triggers.

Rimming

I don't know that there are many people I would tell this to, but having my part-ner's mouth on my ass is so pleasurable I can hardly stand it.—Naomi

Analingus, or rimming, is a sex practice that many do not admit to. Yet, the anal area is full of nerve endings, and for many analingus is as pleasurable as other forms of oral sex.

Most people are concerned about the cleanliness of such a practice. If you are interested in rimming your partner, or vice versa, you can first clean up with soap and water. Using a barrier of latex or plastic wrap also protects you from bacteria and STDs. Many who practice anal sex also clean internally by gentle rinsing with soap and water, or an enema. Keep in mind that because of the anatomy of the lower intestine, little feces is found in the rectum or anal canal (see chapter 5). Be careful not to let any lubricant or saliva around the anus drip into the vagi-nal area. The bacteria from the anus can cause a vaginal infection.

The How-to's of Rimming

The anus is a very delicate part of your body, rich in nerve endings, and extremely responsive to touch. You can kiss, lick, and caress. You can nibble the flesh sur-rounding the anus. With arousal, the anus will open, and you'll be able to fit more of your tongue inside. If your partner is a woman, make sure that you do not move from her anus to her vagina. Take care to prevent vaginal infections.

- Kiss and lick the belly, back, butt, and inner thighs. Let your partner antic-ipate the pleasure to come.
- Nibble at the flesh surrounding the anus.
- Blow warm air gently across the anus.
- Grab a dental dam or other barrier and put a dab of lube on your partner's side.
- Circle the anus with the tip of your tongue.
- Press your tongue flat against the anus and let your partner enjoy the heat and pressure.

- Gently insert the tip of your tongue into the anus.
- Pull out a latex glove and some lube. With a woman partner, you can insert a finger into her vagina as your tongue penetrates her anus. With a man, you can gently stroke his penis as you attend to his anus.

Safer Oral Sex

Through oral sex you can exchange many a bodily fluid. Semen, including pre-come, and blood from menstruation are two of the bodily fluids with the highest concentrations of HIV. The risk factor in contacting vaginal secretions (with no blood) is fairly low. The tissues of the anus, mouth and gums, and vagina can have tiny tears that allow sexually transmitted diseases to pass.

Assess your risk based on your sexual behaviors and HIV status, as well as your partner's. To practice safer fellatio, you can use a condom. Try putting a spot of water-based lubricant inside the tip of the condom to help it slide and increase stimulation for your partner. Remember to hold onto the tip as you put on the condom so air won't be trapped in the tip, which may cause breakage. There are condoms made of alternative materials for those allergic to latex. Lambskin condoms are not effective for preventing the transmission of HIV.

For cunnilingus, you can purchase dental dams, which are squares of latex used in dental procedures, or you can cut open a condom or latex glove and use it as a barrier. To use a condom, cut off the tip, then snip it up one side, opening it into a square. Likewise, you can cut open a glove by snipping off the fingers and up one side. If you use dental dams or cut-open condoms or gloves, mark one side with a pen so that if you slip, you'll know which side goes where. My favorite is plastic food wrap. When using plastic wrap, rip off a long piece and wrap it underneath and around you. No hands! Plastic wrap is also a good substitute for those who are sensitive to latex. A dab of water-based lubricant on the recipient's side of the barrier increases sensitivity.

Remember to use a latex barrier for rimming as well. Again, place some lubricant on the receiver's side of the barrier, and go to town!

Sex Guide Exercises

1. How do you feel after reading this chapter? What do you notice in your thinking, emotions, and sensations?

2. Take out a mirror and look at your own genitals, the area where your partner will be up close and personal during oral sex. Look at the colors, feel the textures. This is a whole and healthy part of you. What do you appreciate about your genitals? Make a list of ten things.

3. What do you like and dislike about oral sex? Specifically, what do you like most and least about cunnilingus? Fellatio? Rimming? Talk with someone about what you like and dislike.

4. What did you discover about yourself in reading this chapter?

chapter ten

Penetration

There are all kind of ways to enjoy penetration. You certainly can enjoy vaginal or anal intercourse with a penis—or a dildo. You can also enjoy fingers, vibrators, and even your partner's whole hand.

Penetration is not limited to your vagina. Many women (and men) enjoy anal penetration—with fingers, vibrators, butt plugs, dildos, and hands.

Most women do not reach orgasm from vaginal or anal penetration alone, but need some form of clitoral stimulation. The same is true for men; very few men reach orgasm from anal penetration without some form of penile stimulation.

There are all kinds of ways to enjoy penetration, both when being penetrated and when penetrating your partner. This chapter will explore some of your options.

Vaginal Penetration

There are numerous ways to enjoy vaginal penetration. You may like being penetrated with your own or your partner's fingers, or with a dildo, either in your partner's or your own hand, or strapped on with a harness. You may like your partner's penis best. Maybe you prefer your partner's fingers or hand, which can stimulate places that a penis might not reach, like the G-spot.

You'll notice different sensations at different depths of the vagina. The nerves nearer the opening of the vaginal passage tend to be more sensitive to and stimulated by movement. The deeper part of the vaginal passage responds more readily to pressure. Many woman find the cervix sensitive to touch and pressure, some liking the sensation and others finding it uncomfortable. Where do you feel the most pleasure in your vagina? Are there different sensations and depths that you like?

The G-Spot

The G-spot is spoken of by tantra practitioners (see chapter 15) as the "sacred spot" or a center of concentrated sexual intensity for many women. Tantra practitioners also speak of the G-spot as an area that holds sexual trauma. Many survivors have told me that working with the G-spot has been central in healing and releasing past sexual trauma. Some survivors report intense vulnerability, tears, or rage when having their G-spot stimulated.

> I felt so vulnerable and opened up. I did not know that she was stimulating my G-spot. I was not familiar with that at the time. It really sent me to another level, out there. Afterward I cried and shook and felt cleansed somehow.—Akaya

As discussed in chapter 5, on anatomy, some women ejaculate with G-spot stimulation. Although not all women experience G-spot ejaculation, there are techniques that can help you learn how, if you're interested. Allow yourself plenty of time to explore your G-spot and discover what arouses you. Urinate before you begin. When you are about to ejaculate, you may feel like you need to pee; you can dissipate this fear by knowing you just went. Also G-spot stimulation can cause bladder infections in some women; you can help to prevent this by urinating before and after you play. If you feel the sensation of having to pee when you come, bear down to release the ejaculate. Please note that this can be a very wet ordeal. You may want to have towels close by.

You can stimulate your own G-spot with your fingers or a firm dildo. Some dildos are curved especially to reach the G-spot. Your partner can stimulate your

G-spot with a hand or a dildo. Tell your partner where the sensation feels most intense and what you want. Many woman also like to have their clitoris stimulated at the same time. Try touching your clit, having your partner touch you, or using a vibrator while your G-spot is being stimulated.

> I have learned how to ejaculate. It took patience and time. It was actually a great way to get to know my genitals and sexual responses. It is wet and fun...kind of intense in a different way.—Daren

Hands and Fisting

Lots of folks get freaked out at the idea of fisting. The term *fisting* can sound aggressive or violent when taken out of context. But it simply refers to inserting a whole hand into the vagina. Fisting has nothing to do with punching the vagina. The term comes from the fact that once a hand is fully inserted, it naturally curls up into an fist, given the amount of room available.

Believe it? Well, it is not so hard to believe when you know women's anatomy. Vaginal membrane is extremely pliable and sturdy. After all, whole babies pass through there. Think back to the information in chapter 5 on women's sexual response cycle. When a woman is sexually aroused, the vaginal walls open and lubricate, and the uterus lifts upward, creating a large ballooned area at the end of the vaginal passage near the cervix. There is enough space in there for a hand (depending, of course, upon both the size of the hand and the woman's anatomy).

Fisting requires relaxation and trust on the receiver's end—plus a high degree of sexual arousal. It usually helps to have ongoing clitoral stimulation while fisting. Fisting is an intense sensation by most accounts. Many survivors report a response similar to that caused by G-spot stimulation, with the release of trauma and emotions.

> The first time my lover and I were successful at fisting, I cried and cried. It wasn't that it hurt, or caused any particular emotional pain. It felt like a release, almost a relief really.—Stephanie

Here are the how-to's of fisting: Get out your water-based lubricant, and play sexually until you are well aroused. (Remember: never use oil-based lubricant in the vagina.) Insert fingers one or two at a time until there is plenty of room for all four. The idea is to make your hand as skinny as possible. Tuck your thumb into the fold of your fingers and fold the two sides of your hand as close together as possible. Your knuckles should face the posterior or back side of the vaginal passage.

The partner being fisted is in charge all the way. Listen to her words and her body. If you are being fisted, communicate and above all, relax. Bring your breath into your pelvis and let it relax and open. Go slowly. If you are doing the fisting, let your partner slowly press down onto your hand.

Getting the width of the knuckles through the narrow passage of your pelvic bones is the part where most first-timers turn back. *Use lots of lube.* I could say that five more times. When you are ready, your partner can ease his or her knuckles inside by slowly rotating the hand past the pubic bone. For the fistee, this is a good time to take a deep breath and exhale with the entrance. This may be painful until you find the proper route through. Some folks twist in, turning the hand palm up once they are in. The fister's hand will curl up into a fistlike shape; thus the name. Stop if any part is too painful. Once in, you can slowly turn the hand, move it gently up and down, or gently move in and out.

> I discovered that my greatest pleasure is in fisting. I love to have my hand inside a woman's vagina, to feel everything she feels. I love to take her inside of me. To feel filled, overwhelmed by the fucking.—Max

Fisting can be incredibly intimate and evoke vulnerably in both you and your partner. Respect this in your play.

The How-to's of Vaginal Penetration

There is so much more to vaginal penetration than athletic thrusting, though once aroused, many women love to be penetrated deeply and firmly. Tell your partner what feels best, or ask her what *she* likes. Remember to communicate and enjoy the exploration.

Whether you're receiving your lover's penis or dildo, or penetrating your female partner, the following are some places to begin. You can share these suggestions with your partner or try them out yourself:

- Tug gently at the pubic hairs.
- Put your whole hand over her vulva; feel the heat and pressure.
- Lightly tap or slap the vulva with your hand.
- Snap on a glove, grab the lube, and trace the opening of her vagina with your fingers.
- Put a condom on your partner's penis—or invite your partner to put a condom on your dildo.
- Run the head of the penis or dildo all around the vulva without entering.
- Enter the vagina only an inch or two, and move in and out.
- Move your hips in a steady motion, then move in circles.
- Have your partner insert two or three fingers into your vagina, and twist and turn his or her hand while thrusting.
- Enter the vagina shallowly and then deeply.
- Put your fingers into her vagina and stimulate her G-spot with a "come-hither" motion.
- Look at your partner.
- Move your body, breathe, and relax.

Anal Penetration

Anal sex is coming into its own these days. While historically it has found its place on the kinky side of the ledger, anal sex is becoming mainstream. At Good Vibrations, I was initially surprised by how many people came in seeking anal sex information and toys. Both men and women were looking for ways to enjoy their butts.

> I find anal sex warm and intense. I get embarrassed talking about it, given the stigma, but I'm getting braver.—MB

I fantasize about anal sex and love it when my lovers touch me there. I can't ask for it yet, though. I am too embarrassed and it brings up memories of my stepfather.—Laura

The anus is a sensitive and nerve-packed area, and it can offer you an enjoyable addition to your sexual pleasure. When playing with the anus, it is important to follow a couple of rules. Always use water-based lubricant for anal penetration. Unlike the vagina, the anus does not produce its own lubrication. To protect the sensitive skin within the anal canal, and to make the experience enjoyable for the recipient, you must use lubrication. Relax. Anal sex will not be successful if you are tense. Breathe. Let the muscles around your butt and pelvis relax.

When practicing anal sex, the person on the receiving end should control the speed and depth of penetration. Communicate with your partner about how it's going.

You can enjoy anal penetration with fingers and hands, with a penis, or with sex toys, such as a dildo or butt plug. Tristan Taormino, author of *The Ultimate Guide to Anal Sex for Women*, writes, "Never poke the anus; instead, stroke the opening with the pad of your finger." Ease your way inside the anus by caressing the opening with your finger. The sphincter muscles will automatically close if you try to penetrate by poking straight into the anus.

If you are using anything other than what is attached to your body to penetrate the ass—like a dildo or butt plug—make sure it is flanged at the bottom. This means that the bottom of the toy widens into a broad base to prevent it from slipping up into the anal canal and beyond. Unlike the vaginal canal, the anus leads right into the body. An unflanged toy could slip up into the large intestines. This is very painful and dangerous, not to mention embarrassing, and can result in a trip to the nearest emergency room.

Again, many people are concerned about cleanliness when practicing anal sex. Before engaging in anal sex you can wash yourself with soapy water or use an enema to cleanse the anal canal. If you are planning to have anal sex, be careful about what you eat. Stay away from hot or spicy foods and small seeds, like those on strawberries or in kiwis. These are not digested and can scrape the sensitive lining of the anal area.

Some people also practice anal fisting, or handballing, which takes great care because of the sensitivity of the membrane lining the anal canal. The process is similar to vaginal fisting. If you are interested in anal fisting, read up on anal sex and anal anatomy first. It is best to learn from someone with experience.

Male Prostate

In men, the prostate gland can be stimulated through anal penetration (see chapter 5 for more on the prostate). Many men find prostate stimulation very pleasurable, though, as with G-spot stimulation in women, it may be too intense or painful for some men. The prostate can be reached by inserting a finger or toy about three inches into the anus and pressing toward the front of the body, using that old come-hither motion again.

The How-to's of Anal Penetration

Anal penetration requires even more communication than other sexual activities. The anus and rectum are fragile. Approach with care. If you prefer toys to fingers or a penis, pick a slender dildo for starters. Remember to use a lot of lubricant for anal play. And keep anal bacteria out of the vagina. You can place a bunched-up a sheet or towel over the vagina to catch any drips of lube if you are being penetrated from behind.

Whether you're penetrating your partner or receiving your lover's penis or dildo, the following are some ideas to try. You can share these suggestions with your partner or try them out yourself:

- Tug at his or her pubic hairs.
- Caress your partner's genitals, thighs, and butt.
- Use your fingers to become familiar with your partner's body.
- Snap on a glove, grab the lube, and trace the opening of the anus with your fingers.
- Massage the opening of the anus.
- Make sure your partner is well aroused and open before you insert a finger or toy.

- Use a sweeping motion to enter; don't poke.
- Stimulate the clitoris or stroke the penis as you play.
- Put a condom on your partner's penis or dildo.
- Run the head of your penis or dildo all around the opening without entering.
- Enter slowly; let your partner guide you.
- Penetrate slowly at first. Communicate about the depth and speed.
- Relax, move, and breathe.

Safer Penetration

As with oral sex, you can exchange many bodily fluids through penetration. Semen, including pre-come, and blood from menstruation are two of the bodily fluids with the highest concentration of HIV. The risk factor for contact with vaginal secretions (no blood) is fairly low. Anal penetration often causes tiny tears in the sensitive anal tissues, allowing for the transmission of blood and other bodily fluids. If you practice anal sex, practice it safely with latex barriers.

To practice safer sex during vaginal penetration, use a condom on your partner's penis or dildo, or a latex glove on your partner's hand. Again, using a bit of water-based lubricant in the tip of the condom will help it slide and increase stimulation. Remember to hold onto the tip as you put on the condom to prevent air from being trapped at the tip, which can cause breakage. There are condoms made of alternative materials for those allergic to latex. Lambskin condoms are not effective for preventing the transmission of HIV.

When using latex gloves, get a size that fits you snugly. This will increase the sensitivity. Slather the glove with water-based lube and you are set to go.

Just another reminder regarding your genital health: Do not bring a toy or hand from the anus back to the vulva without washing it first, or replacing the glove or condom. The bacteria from the anal area can cause an infection in the vagina.

Penetration and Triggers

Penetration can be triggering for many survivors. If you were vaginally or anally penetrated during the abuse, you may find it painful or upsetting to have vaginal or anal sex now.

For some survivors, penetration can be painful, because tension and trauma are held in the pelvic region, or because of an infection or other medical problem. If you have vaginal or anal pain during penetration, go to a skilled medical practitioner to get it checked out. Some survivors have gotten sexually transmitted diseases from the sexual abuse or unsafe sexual practices. Vaginismus, fibroid tumors, and vaginal infections can cause pain during penetration. Some survivors will have scarring within the vagina from severe abuse.

Trauma caused by sexual abuse that included penetration can be held throughout the pelvic area as tension, pain, and/or numbness. As you work with this area of your body, releasing the pain, memories, and trauma, your sensations may change. Many survivors have this experience.

> *The feelings in my hips and genitals changed as I healed. I used to feel pain and tension when I had sex, or I wouldn't feel much at all, as if I didn't have any nerve endings in that part of my body. As I have thawed that part of me, lots of feelings of pain, fear, and anger have come out. It's as if they were stored in there under some sheath of ice until I could feel them.—Jenifer*

When working with triggers related to penetration, take it slowly. Pay attention to what comes up throughout your pelvic area. This can be one of the most loaded areas of the body for survivors and one of the most potent for healing.

You may find it useful to control the depth and speed of the penetration during sex. Communicate with your partner throughout the sexual experience, telling him or her when to slow down, when to speed up, and how deeply to enter you. It is usually easier to control the depth and speed of penetration if you are on top. Some folks find it embarrassing to talk all the way through a sexual encounter, yet it can greatly add to your pleasure and sense of connection.

Check in visually with your partner as well. What is it like to look at your partner during penetration? Keeping your eyes open may also help you stay in the present and not slip back into the past. Notice your partner and your surroundings, breathe, and feel your sensations and body. You can remain connected to yourself this way, which will keep you resourceful and able to choose how to respond to a trigger.

Changing positions can also be useful when you feel triggered during penetration. For some, lying on their stomach while being penetrated from behind is triggering, while being on top is not. You can also try facing each other, lying side by side, or the spoons position. You can both sit up, legs wrapped around each other, for another variation. Exploring is the name of the game. What positions helps you stay in your body? In which positions do you feel the most resourceful and empowered?

Penetration need not be a trigger forever. If you want a particular sexual option, you can work with the trigger using the resources and exercises in this book. The choice is yours as to what sexual options you want to have. The next chapter will guide you through ways to heal through your triggers.

Sex Guide Exercises

1. How do you feel after reading this chapter? What do you notice in your thinking, emotions, and sensations?
2. What do like most and least about penetration? Specifically, what do you like and dislike about vaginal penetration? Anal penetration? Penetration with sex toys? Fingers and hands? Talk with someone else about what you like and dislike.
3. What did you discover about yourself in reading this chapter?

chapter eleven

Embracing Triggers

If you arrange your sex life to avoid triggers, you'll end up with no room left for your sex life.—Stephanie

Many survivors feel understandably frustrated when it comes to triggers. You may be in a stage of sexual recovery in which you are dealing with them all the time. You may be so triggered sexually that you do not want to be sexual at all. Most survivors just want to get rid of triggers altogether.

In this chapter, I want to introduce a different approach. What if triggers were not to be avoided but rather explored, felt, and healed? What if triggers were flags waving as if to say, "Hey, over here, there is something needing healing and attention"? Triggers are healable. You need not assume that because oral sex triggers you now, it always will. Once you have released the trauma from the area of your body where the trigger is stored and processed the experience emotionally, the trigger will fade.

The intent in this work is to heal your sexuality to such an extent that you can fully make your own choices about sex. You get to choose your sexual expression based upon your own needs and desires, not those limits and traumas induced by childhood sexual abuse. This chapter tells you how to achieve this healing through your triggers.

What Is a Trigger?

Triggers are automatic responses connected to your past sexual abuse that can suddenly rush into the present. Certain acts, smells, words—perhaps even a tone of voice—can act as triggers that bring up images and feelings from the past. When you are in the middle of being triggered, it may be difficult to distinguish between the past and the present.

> *I've never been one of those survivors who got triggered in the grocery store. My triggers are mostly connected to people and being close. Sex especially triggers me. Many times when having sex, images of my father will come rushing in and I can no longer tell the difference between him and my lover. I get terrified and shut down, then just try to hurry up and get sex over with. It's awful.—Carla*

Triggers seem to arise unexpectedly. They can evoke images or memories of the abuse, emotions, or feelings in your body. Many survivors report being overwhelmed by a sense of not wanting their partner to touch them, or pulling away from physical or sexual touch out of an automatic fear that they will be hurt or betrayed.

> *Sometimes my girlfriend reaches to touch me and I want to push her away. I don't want her near me and I feel nauseated.—Kathy*

Triggers can also be sudden moods that seem to take over. You may be enjoying flirting or talking sexy with your partner and suddenly find yourself angry and annoyed, or grief-stricken. These are typical experiences for survivors.

> *I get so angry, I feel sorry for my husband. We'll be acting playful, flirting, and beginning to be sexual, and I will turn on him. I kind of flip inside. Suddenly I am agitated and annoyed. Everything he does grates on me.—Rona*

Just being confronted with certain sexual acts, smells, sounds, and colors may act as triggers for survivors. Even enjoying certain sexual acts or orgasm may serve as a trigger point.

> *Oral sex…I just can't do it yet. I try, but I start to gag and I feel like I'm that little girl again with my uncle shoving himself down my throat.—Tracy*

I used to cry every time I had an orgasm. I didn't understand it until I remembered the incest. The tears are a mix of relief and guilt and shame. It really stirs up the part of the abuse that physically felt good and all the shame of thinking it was my fault. —Roslyn

Triggers are history seeping through into the present, pieces of memory emerging from the past. While the pain, anger, or confusion can seem to be a response to something that is happening today, it is really a fragment of visual, emotional, or body memory making its way to the surface. Triggers act like cracks in present-day reality that open to unresolved trauma from the past.

Map to Recovery

The same or similar triggers often recur until that piece of memory or trauma is processed and released. In this way, triggers act as flags to alert you to aspects of healing that need to be addressed. Triggers can serve as a map to your recovery and sexual healing. By attending to and healing *through* your triggers, you can unpack the baggage of sexual abuse from your sexuality.

I always used to get triggered by my girlfriend kissing me in a certain way; it made me want to push her away or totally dissociate. I then had the memory of my brother kissing me that same way when he abused me. I cried and got angry and dealt with that memory, and that trigger is put to rest. —Kay

So, what triggers you? What sights, smells, places, sexual positions, or sounds can trigger you? What ways of being sexual make you want to run, dissociate, freeze, or get angry or sad? How about sex and intimacy combined? What happens for you then? Discovering your triggers is like finding important clues on a treasure hunt. This information is vital in the sexual healing process.

Just as you tracked patterns of dissociation in chapter 3, you can track patterns in your triggers. What triggers you sexually? Your own intensity? That you like anal sex, S/M, or other "unacceptable" turn-ons?

I've found that one of my biggest triggers is how intense I can get sexually. I want to fuck, and bite, and grab. It is all consensual, we are adults, and I still get triggered into this feeling of shame.—Jeanie

Note how your body changes when you are triggered. What sensations do you notice? What happens in your body? Do you stop breathing, hold your jaws tight, tighten your genitals or sphincter muscle? How do your moods and emotions shift?

What recurring images, sounds, memories, emotions, or body sensations emerge when you are triggered? Explore your triggers; there is a world of information to gain.

Not having sex triggers me. I start to get all weird, like I am unworthy, unloved. I feel like I need to go find a trick or one-night stand to prove myself again.—Lourdes

Saying "no" is an unbelievable trigger for me. I either can't say it at all, or I start shaking and muttering…I feel like I am five again. My "no" has been incested out of me.—Mimi

Embracing Triggers: This Way Out

The idea of embracing your triggers may seem counterintuitive at first. You may feel uncomfortable and unsettled with this way of dealing with triggers, yet I have seen its effectiveness time and time again. Instead of avoiding and moving away from triggers, you can begin to move toward and into them. When you get triggered you can say, "Hey, good news, I am triggered. Now I can free up more of me!" When you move yourself toward and into a trigger, you have the opportunity to then process the material and move through it. In doing this you can release the trigger from your body, emotions, and mind and be complete with it. Triggers act as signposts to what is in need of healing. They guide you on the road to freedom.

Tracking Triggers

A. *I get triggered when* (sights, sounds, smells, positions, places)...

I really let go and get into sex. If I like or love sex, then I must have wanted the abuse.

My husband comes at me from behind.

I am awoken in the middle of the night to have sex. I can't tell where I am or who my boyfriend is.

The inside of my right thigh is stroked repeatedly. I want to kick.

My legs or arms are held down.

My nipples are touched softly. This unnerves me; I need a firmer touch.

I see men who look like my uncle.

B. *What happens in my body is* (sensations)...

I get extremely tense between my shoulder blades.

My breathing gets really shallow.

My feet and the lower part of my body seem far away, not quite a part of me anymore.

My genitals and anus tense up.

I float out of my body.

My throat gets tight and I feel like I can't speak.

C. *Recurring visuals, smells, sounds, emotions and body memories are*...

This picture of my dad entering my bedroom and coming toward me.

A picture of my grandpa with a hard-on.

Being penetrated from behind; this grips my body and senses.

The smell of his deodorant.

The smell of alcohol on his breath.

Having weight on top of me, which makes me feel panicked and trapped.

The sound of their voices; I don't know where to run.

Most of us hate triggers and getting triggered. They can be painful, annoying, and devastating, and they interrupt otherwise good experiences. Because of this, many survivors try to avoid triggers as much as possible. They try to organize their lives, and especially their sex lives, to avoid the uncomfortable and often painful feelings that being triggered can bring up. Eventually, people can a build a narrow life entirely motivated by avoiding triggers.

Sex triggered me so much that I eventually avoided it altogether. I tried to become asexual and rid myself of all notions of being erotic. This has cost me a lot of joy in my life.—Mimi

You know, in taking on recovering from all this stuff, I realized that I had not touched myself in years. This is so sad when I think about it now. They scared me away from my own body.—Maria

Triggers are funny creatures. When they are avoided, they seem to become bigger or more powerful, while the space for *you* becomes smaller. Avoiding triggers also leaves all of the land mines of sexual abuse in place, so the terrain of your life continues to feel dangerous and untrustworthy. When triggers are taken on, felt, and processed, they shrink or transform altogether. What was once a trigger becomes a completed part of your history. You may notice it periodically, but it no longer runs you.

I didn't think I would ever make it to the place where I could enjoy sex and not be triggered. It is amazing to me that I have arrived. I still deal with a trigger periodically, but mostly I am present and enjoying myself. It is great!—Lee

By trying to ignore triggers, you are saying that the trigger is more powerful than you are. This, of course, is not the case. You are more powerful than what happened to you. It may not feel like it sometimes, but I can assure you this is the case. You are more powerful than what happened to you or you would not have made it.

The first time I decided to stay with a trigger to try to process it, I was terrified. I thought it was insane to keep myself there. It was painful, and I cried and remembered new stuff. I hated it, and I got through it. That trigger and those memories were never as scary again.—Melanie

My body would shake whenever I tried to hang with the touch that triggered me the most. But I learned to breathe and just let myself shake. It felt like all the terror and fear of the abuse, all the tears could now pour out of me in a way that they couldn't before. I feel very thankful and compassionate with myself now. —Stephanie

Since I really started taking on my triggers and treating them like messengers of important information, I have been changing. I can masturbate and not check out or have a guilt attack now. No, even more than that, I can masturbate, feel sexy, and enjoy myself.—Halli

Trigger Plan and Tools

So, just how do you handle triggers? What do you do in the midst of being sexual when you are no longer with the living? How can you use your triggers to heal yourself? Before we begin, I suggest that you check out your network of support. Having people you can talk to, cry with, and explore these ideas with is essential to the healing process. If you haven't begun to gather a support network, please do so now. You can find advice on this in chapter 1.

The following are simple steps to take when you are triggered in a sexual situation. These tools can be used in both partner sex and masturbation. I suggest that you review these steps first in a nonsexual situation. Give them a test run. Talk them through with a friend, partner, or counselor, or write about them in your journal. Practicing these steps outside of a sexual encounter will make them much easier to use while being sexual. It is hard to try a new approach when you are feeling triggered in the middle of sex. By practicing these tools first, you will have resources at hand to help you through.

These steps are encapsulated in the Trigger Plan later in this chapter. This is an easy format to use in preparing yourself.

NOTICE.

Begin by noticing when you are triggered. This can be the biggest step. What is triggering you? What sensations are you feeling in your body? Are you breathing? Often we blame our partners for the discomfort, irritation, or dislike that emerges with a trigger. Thoroughly check out the source of your uneasiness with your partner when it comes up. Are you triggered? How can your partner be an ally to you now, instead of an enemy? As with dissociation, your partner can help you notice when you are triggered.

STOP AND BREATHE.

Stop, pause, and breathe. Assess the situation. What are you feeling? What's going on? What do you need? It is fine to take a break in the middle of sex. Stopping and addressing the trigger will ultimately make your sexual experience more satisfying, safe, and healing. Refer to your internal sensations of safety or your emotional resource (see chapter 1).

CHOOSE.

Now is your opportunity. Once you have noticed your trigger and paused, there are numerous options for handling it. You'll find some options listed below, under Many Choices. Please add to the list those particular things that work for you. When making a choice as how to handle a trigger, check in with what you need right now and what will be best for your ongoing healing process. If in the past you have tended to choose to stop being sexual, try something different instead. Take a break and then re-engage sexually. Or change what you are doing but remain in physical contact with yourself or your partner. If you have consistently tried to push through triggers, now try stopping. Attend to the child in you. Or move toward the trigger to work with it. Taking new risks is important. It expands your options and lets you learn to do what was previously not possible.

ENGAGE.

Continue to be present with yourself and your sex partner. Communicate your choice and talk it over with her or him. Then, engage. Keep bringing yourself to the experience, whether you have chosen to go into the trigger, to continue being sexual, or to get up and go on a walk. Stay connected to yourself, your body, and your partner as much as possible. This is a process of retraining your body. You can be in contact with yourself and another even if you are triggered. You don't have to go away or disappear. You can stay in your body and at choice. If your first choice doesn't work for you, feel free to change your mind and make a different choice.

RETURN.

Go back to the beginning and start again as necessary.

Many Choices

Building a whole repertoire of choices gives you numerous avenues you can take when triggered. A generous array of options also allows you to choose different approaches at different times. You may be best supported in your healing process by stopping sex altogether in one encounter, and best served by continuing in another. There are no hard-and-fast rules about what to do when you are triggered. Watch for patterns in your response to triggers. If you always do the same thing, such as stopping sex or trying to go around the trigger, try other approaches. Building options and choices is bringing back into sex what was taken away by sexual abuse.

A number of options follow. This is a limited list; please add to it other options that work for you.

Go into the Trigger

You can choose to go into the trigger by keeping your focus and attention on the visual, auditory, or bodily sensations that have been triggered. Keep breathing and stay open to feeling your emotions and the sensations in your body. You can continue to do the thing that initially triggered you, to help take you further into it. Go there gently. The intention behind this choice is to move into, feel, remember, release, and complete the stored memory or trauma. You may move into grieving, anger, fear, or some other emotion connected to the abuse. Let those feelings emerge and be released. When going into a trigger, physically expressing the emotions it brings up is a powerful tool and can move you through it more quickly.

If you are with your partner, share with her or him what is happening and how you are feeling. Let your emotions and body release. If you are shaking, crying, or laughing, do it fully. If you need to express anger, yell into a pillow, hit the bed, or twist a towel as hard as you can. (For more information on safe ways to express traumatic emotions, see chapter 12).

If you are experiencing a memory of abuse, tell your partner as much as you can about it. When you are able to make eye contact with your partner, do so. Connect with his or her support in the present.

The only rule during the expressing of intense emotions is not to hurt yourself or anyone else. Do not break or ruin any object that is important to you or anyone else. I find that while most survivors are afraid that they might hurt some-one or get out of control if they express the pain, they actually tend to err on the side of holding in their emotions. For most survivors, having feelings, especially those related to the abuse, was dangerous as a child. But now you have the oppor-tunity to feel and express what you could not before. Grief, rage, terror, and con-fusion are all completely appropriate responses to sexual abuse.

If you choose to move into the trigger and you are with a partner, first make sure that both of you are ready and willing to go there. This can be an intense experience for your partner as well. During the preparation of your trigger plan, or as you choose to go into the trigger, tell your partner what you need. Do you need to be held? Do you need your partner to back off while you get angry? Communicate your needs as much as possible to help you both move through the experience as smoothly as possible.

If you are alone and decide to go into a trigger, make contact with someone else afterward by phone or a visit. Tell someone what you went through. Share how you are. Reconnect with another human being. This step is essential to take you out of isolation and rebuild connection and relationship with others.

Once you have released the emotion, look inside to reestablish a sense of well-being. As discussed in chapter 1, you can build a sense of internal safety through somatic practice. You'll learn more about creating internal resources in chapter 12. For now, consciously notice that though you are feeling pain, you are okay. Nothing bad has happened. You are healing.

Watch from a Distance

Another approach to being with a trigger is to watch it from a distance, while remaining rooted in the present. This can be useful with a trigger you have already processed or a trigger you are working on but don't want to process fully right now. Noticing objects in the room, colors on the walls, sounds in the environment will help you remain rooted in the present. Note these out loud if you need to. Feel your body—your weight on the bed or your form filling the chair. Remind yourself of the year and the current date, and that you are here in the present. Breathe. From the present, attend to the trigger or memory.

Acknowledge it by speaking about it out loud or writing it down. This approach acknowledges the trigger without moving into it fully. You may want to work with this trigger at another time in a nonsexual setting.

MOVE

A great way to work with being triggered is to get up and move. Walk around, stretch, breathe, and relax your body. You can also make sounds or shake your body to "shake off" the trigger. Moving can have the effect of bringing you to a present and settled place in which you can return to being sexual.

TAKE CARE OF THE CHILD

You can approach a trigger as if it were a small child who is afraid and upset. Treat the trigger as you would a real child who interrupted you while you were having sex. Stop being sexual for the moment and attend to the little girl or inner child. What does she need? Pick her up and comfort her; sit down and rock her. You can use a doll or stuffed animal to represent her, if that will make it easier. Explain to her that sex is for grown-ups, not for kids. Once you have taken care of her, put her back to bed. You can then return to sex if you so chose.

LET'S MAKE A DEAL

Engaging in internal negotiations with triggers is another approach. You can "talk to" triggers as if they were parts of you that could communicate. You can ask the triggered part of yourself what it needs and how you might provide that. You will often find that the trigger is a cry for love and attention. You can negotiate to take care of that triggered part of yourself at a later date. If that seems agreeable, make a specific date and time when you will check in with yourself again and attend to the trigger. Keep your commitment.

CHANGE SEXUAL ACTIVITIES

Changing positions or sexual activities, turning on the light, or adjusting your environment can shift a trigger for you. If you are uncomfortable or feel uneasy with what you are doing, communicate this to your partner and adjust accordingly. This can add to your sexual play and does not need to be a distraction that ends the encounter.

There are innumerable sexual activities to choose from. If what you are doing is triggering, change activities. If the weight of your partner on top of you triggers you, get on top yourself. Try sitting up or lying side by side. If your partner is sucking on your breasts in a way that triggers you, ask her to kiss your stomach instead. Or turn over onto your stomach and have him lie on your back. Here's an opportunity to get creative. Satisfying sex rarely follows the first-through-fourth-base model of lovemaking.

If you are having a hard time staying present with your partner, open your eyes and look at him or her. Try changing rooms if need be, or bring objects into the space that remind you of your safety and empowerment.

Go to the Movies

You can also choose to change activities altogether. You can choose something that is still sensual or erotic, such as massage with no genital contact, feeding each other foods you like, or bathing together. Or, you can take a break from sex altogether. Take a walk, listen to music, draw, go to the movies, pet your dog—whatever you like. Whatever your choice, practice being embodied and present with yourself and your partner.

Return to the Present

Pause and breathe. Orient yourself to the present by noticing objects, sounds, smells, temperatures, and sensations. Remind yourself where you are, whom you are with, and that what you are doing is consensual. Remind yourself that right now you are powerful and at choice. Review the reasons you like to be sexual and how expressing yourself sexually benefits you. Return to the present and continue to be sexual.

Change the Story

Once you have worked with acknowledging, feeling, and gaining information from your triggers, you can work with changing the story. If a visual memory or body memory arises, you can intercede and imagine a different outcome.

Let's say the body memory of being trapped or held down is triggered. You can stop, breathe, and then imagine pushing off of you the person who is holding you down. Then imagine running for help. Your current adult self can swoop in, pick up the abuser, and throw him across the room, while whisking your frightened child self away to safety. You can imagine that an ally comes in and stops the abuse, telling you that this will never happen again.

This is an opportunity to get creative. You can rewrite the story in any way you choose. Now, as an adult, you are able to respond to the trigger, take control of the situation, and take back your power and innocence. Make sure the ending of your story includes getting you (and your little girl) to a safe place where there is support.

Say "No" to Repeating Triggers

What if the trigger persists after you've processed it emotionally? Some triggers seem to return out of habit more than anything else. If a recurring image or trigger appears, you can tell it, "No, you are no longer welcome here. Do not come back." You can decide now who is allowed in your inner space and what is going to happen there. This is a process of setting internal boundaries, which you are now in control of. Turn away the image or trigger each time it appears, until it doesn't return again.

> I had this repeating image of my father that would come to me when I got really turned on. His face would appear and somehow want to be a part of the turn-on. I finally just yelled at him. I told him to get out, and that he was not allowed here anymore. I sent the image out into space, making it smaller and smaller until it disappeared. I did this every time that his face appeared, until it didn't happen anymore. It was great, like taking back my own space.—Anne

Your Creations

Take a moment now to come up with other ways that you can heal through and work with your triggers. As you practice using these tools, you will get more skilled at handling your triggers, and the process will go more quickly. You can use these tools while masturbating or when having sex with a partner.

Trigger Plan

Developing a trigger plan is like preparing for a trip. You usually choose your itinerary and gather your maps before you buy your plane ticket. Similarly, set up your trigger plan before you are in a sexual setting. You can develop this plan to use on your own, without necessarily letting your sexual partner in on it. But sharing the plan with your sexual partner can be an empowering risk as well as a great support when working on sexual healing. Please use this plan when being sexual with yourself as well as during partner sex, because masturbation can be just as triggering.

1. Notice.

What are some of your current triggers? What happens when you are triggered? How can you (or your partner) notice that you are triggered? Be specific about behaviors. List at least three signals or signs that let you know you are triggered. For example: I start to get angry and my lover's touch bugs me. I hold my breath. I want to say something, but I feel like I can't. I worry that I will hurt my lover's feelings. Then I start tensing up in my body and find myself just "bearing it," waiting for the whole thing to be over.

2. Stop.

Take a deep breath. Stop the sexual activity. You can do this by using a safeword, by moving your body to communicate that you need to stop, or by getting up to go to the bathroom. Breathe again. Name three things you can do to stop sexual activity when you are triggered. Refer to your sense of internal safety and resources.

3. Choose.

Now you get to choose how you would like to proceed. Keep breathing. Relax your body. It is easiest to do this step if you have already generated a list of options you feel will work for you. Choose from this list what will meet your needs and support your sexual healing now.

4. Engage.

Instead of dissociating, engage in whatever strategy you have decided on. Continue to build your capacity to stay present and tolerate the sensations and feelings that are a part of this healing work. Just a reminder: you are always allowed to change your mind and to choose again. If you find that you consistently make the same choice, try choosing something different. For instance, if you usually choose to calm the trigger and continue being sexual, try going into the trigger instead. If you consistently choose to stop being sexual, practice continuing slowly. Bring yourself to your own edge of discomfort so that you can expand your possibilities and process the abuse.

5. Return.

Go back to the beginning whenever you need to.

Tell It Like It Is: Communication and Triggers

Triggers provide a great opportunity to communicate clearly. While it can be challenging initially to talk about triggers, your needs, or sex, the ability to do so will greatly improve your sex life and satisfaction, and aid your healing. Again, it is much easier to communicate in the moment if you have practiced first outside of the vulnerable and high-risk environment of a sexual encounter. Talk about sex and your trigger plan while sitting at the kitchen table, or driving in the car, or taking a walk.

Like many people, your partner might also be uncomfortable talking about sex. The trigger plan is a great way to begin to speak about sex, your choices, and your needs. Depending upon how intimate you are, you can show your trigger plan to your partner, create it together, or choose to share specific parts while keeping others private.

The more you are able to talk to your sexual partners, the more successful you will be at negotiating triggers, dissociation, and/or sexual abuse memories with them as they emerge. In many cases, just telling a partner what is happening can begin to alter the experience. You can then ask your partner for what you need—perhaps to stop or change what he or she is doing. Partners consistently say they would rather be informed about what is going on than feel that something is "off" in the experience, or not know at all. Communicating gives you the option of respecting and taking care of both yourself and your partner.

I don't tell my lover when I am triggered. It is too embarrassing and I just want it all to go away. Instead, I go away. I usually just space out.—Debbie

I am very clear now with my partner when I am triggered. He will often notice me going away before I do. Both of us are committed to having sex only when we are present. So, he'll speak up or I will, and then I have the chance to come back. We'll say, "Oh, it is you. It's you." He is teaching me that the purpose of sex is not sensation. It's connection.—Aurora

Safewords

As you communicate with a partner about sex and triggers, it can be useful to create a safeword, an agreed-upon word that you can use to communicate "Stop, I am triggered," or "Wait, I need to talk about or renegotiate what we are doing." Choose a simple word that you don't usually use during sex. Some people use traffic signal colors: "yellow" means check in or slow down, and "red" means stop. When either of you safewords, all activity is suspended immediately while you check in with each other. Both partners must agree to respect this. Come up with a word that works for you.

Many survivors find it difficult to speak once they are triggered. If this is true for you, you can invent a safeword position or hand signal, such as sitting up or waving your right hand. Again, be creative, and choose something that you can do. Once you have used your safeword or signal, stop and collect yourself. Now is the time to use the trigger plan and decide how to move forward.

Remember that when being sexual, and particularly when dealing with triggers and healing from sexual abuse, both you and your partner are in vulnerable states. Be respectful of yourself as well as of your partner. Take care of your own needs while remembering that your partner is a person with feelings, too. This doesn't mean you should ignore your own needs to take care of your partner's, but that you should communicate as clearly as possible in order to respect both of you.

Troubling Desire

Some survivors have sexual desires that bother them. You may feel like your desires are self-destructive. Self-destructive sexual desires can include disembodied or nonconsensual sex, sex when you are intoxicated or high to the extent that your judgment is impaired, and sex that makes you feel disempowered or used. You may also have desires that feel like a repeat of the sexual abuse. You may be sexually attracted to children or put yourself in dangerous sexual situations.

It was so hard to finally admit to my therapist that I feel some attraction toward kids. I would never touch one, but I had to really deal with this.—Rose

The turn-ons that seem the most problematic are those that become connected to self-hate and self-destructive tendencies. You may be attracted to people who continue to abuse you sexually or physically, or you may self-inflict wounds. Some survivors find that the only way they can become aroused is to feel humiliated. If you have such troubling desires, learning to separate abuse from your arousal is central to your healing.

It seemed like the only men I was attracted to became violent within the first months. I have been raped by a boyfriend and kept going out with him. I cringe when I think of that now. It was all I knew, to be treated like that. It is what I felt I deserved.—Tracy

Treat these troubling or self-destructive desires like triggers. What needs to be healed or faced? How can you move into the pain to transform it?

Healing Triggers Outside of Partner Sex

Proactively working with your triggers outside of sexual encounters is a powerful way to move your sexual healing forward. I encourage you to regularly work with your sexual triggers on your own, in conversation with friends, therapists, people in support groups, and other sources of support. Dealing with sexual triggers exclusively during sex is unfair to your sex life.

You do not need a sexual partner to heal triggers. Many survivors do the majority of their sexual healing and trigger work outside of being sexual with another person. All of the practices in this chapter can be done on your own.

Masturbation is a perfect way to explore your triggers as well as what pleasures you. Most triggers that will emerge during partner sex will emerge during masturbation. Practice being embodied and working with your triggers during masturbation. Note what tools work for you. This gives you powerful groundwork to take into partner sex.

Feeding the Triggers: A Tool for Healing Triggers

This is a very powerful and effective exercise for healing and attending to triggers. Although it might seem daunting at first, once you get the hang of it, it is really quite simple. This exercise can be done alone or with a friend, partner, or therapist whose role will be to facilitate, witness, and be present for the experience.

1. Arrange two pillows or chairs so that they are facing each other. Sit on one. Close your eyes and get in touch with the trigger that you want to work with. Where is it in your body? How does it feel? (e.g., *I feel a constriction in my chest and back*, or *My stomach gets tights and I feel terrified.*) Fully feel the trigger and be clear about where in your body you feel it.

2. Next, let the trigger float out of you onto the pillow across from you, taking some form. It could look like a monster, a little girl, a color or shape. Just let it take shape. An image or sense will appear. Now describe the creature sitting across from you as specifically as you can. What color is it? How large? Does it have a face, a look in its eye?

3. Once you have a clear sense of the representation of the trigger, ask it out loud, "What do you need?"

4. Switch seats, so that you now occupy the creature or symbol's seat. Take a moment to imagine yourself becoming the creature or symbol. What does it feel like to be this creature? Now respond as the creature. Tell "you" in the other chair what it is you need. Speak in "I" statements: "I need," "I want."

5. If the trigger wants you, for example, to die, to quit ignoring it, or to eat all the food in the house, ask it (or have your partner ask it) what purpose that would serve. "If I died, quit ignoring you, or ate all that food, how would that make you feel?" You want to

I found that to really progress in getting my sexuality back, I had to work on it outside of sex. I wrote about it, and I took it, reluctantly at first, to counseling. After awhile another survivor friend and I made up our own two-person group and talked just about sex and sexual healing. We learned new stuff together, did exercises, and gave ourselves homework. Her support made all the difference.—Stephanie

discover the need beneath the need. Continue to ask these questions until you get to the base of the trigger's needs. Most often, the needs at this point will be for love, safety, acceptance, and forgiveness.

6. Once you have discovered the needs of the trigger you are working with, switch seats and become yourself again. Then, as if by magic, evoke an infinite quantity of love, safety, acceptance, and forgiveness, or whatever it is the trigger symbol needs. Feed the creature what it needs until it is fully and completely satisfied. If you find it difficult to imagine yourself feeding the creature to complete satisfaction, then just imagine that it has been fully fed. Know that all triggers can be fed to their complete satisfaction. Different triggers take in this sustenance in different ways: some eat it, others breathe it in or absorb it into their bodies. Still others take it in best as sounds or colors. Be creative and use what works for your trigger creature.

7. Once the trigger is completely satisfied, or you have imagined that it is, sit quietly. Sit in the emptiness or wholeness. Don't fill it with the next problem, or the next trigger; just sit quietly for a few moments. At this point, many triggers will transform in shape and size. Just notice whatever yours does and be with that. When you are ready, complete the exercise by thanking the creature and yourself.

8. Repeat this exercise with the same or different triggers as needed. Because of the depth of childhood sexual abuse, many triggers will need this feeding more than once. Repeated over time, this approach to healing triggers can be amazingly successful. With practice you can also begin to do this exercise in your own mind. It is a handy tool to carry with you.

I learned a version of this exercise from Tsultrim Allione at the Tara Mandala Retreat Center, as a part of the chöd practice, a practice of Tibetan meditation.

Taking a Break from Sex

It can be powerful for survivors to take a break from being sexual for a period of time, particularly if you feel that all you are really good for or loved for is sex. What would it be like to negotiate time off from sex? What would it be like to learn that people love and are attracted to your person rather than what you can do for them sexually?

Times to consider taking a break from sex include the following:

• When you find yourself consistently having sex to fulfill nonsexual needs for closeness and intimacy: *If I just have sex with him or her I can be held.* What about just asking to be held?

- When you are having sex repeatedly "for your partner" even though you don't want to.
- When you have sex of any kind when you don't want to.
- When you have sex when you are dissociated, checked out, or not really "there."
- When sex is the only way that you can feel your body.
- When having sex is the thing that makes you feel worthy.
- When you have sex because you fear being left if you do not.

Having sex for any of these reasons communicates to your body that you are not safe, that you are being abused, that you are only good for sex. This is what childhood sexual abuse teaches you, and not what you want for your sex life now. Now you can communicate something different to yourself and your body. This means taking on different behaviors and different actions.

Having sex with your partner when you don't want to, or having sex because it is the only reason you believe you are worthy or loved, is not the same as sexual abuse, nor are your sexual partners your perpetrators. But having this kind of sex does reinforce the belief that you have no say about sex and that you are not worth loving as a whole being. The pattern continues over and over again.

There was a point when I was compulsive about sex. I decided to declare a moratorium on sexual activity for four months. After two weeks, I thought I was going to die. I was actually convinced that the peak sexual experience of my life was scheduled for those two weeks and that I'd miss it. During this time out, I was able to discover that my arousal was tied to humiliation because of the abuse.—Aurora

You are now responsible for your well-being and for your body and sexuality. What do you want to be telling yourself? What new experiences and possibilities do you want your body to know?

If you are in a partnership and want to negotiate a time away from sex, talk with your partner about it. Talk about what you need and why. Explain what you think you will gain by not being sexual for a time. It helps to acknowledge that sex is an important part of any partnership, that you want to take care of this part of your own life, and that you want to take care of it in your relationship as well.

When negotiating a break from sex, agree upon a specific amount of time. It can be a month, two months, a year—whatever will work for you both.

What do you want to accomplish or work on during this time, individually and in your relationship? How can you be intimate with your partner while taking a break from sex? Talk about your partner's sexual needs. How else can she or he express sexual energy? Masturbation, reading erotic stories, or even writing them are good options. Be creative.

I have found that this is not generally a good time to introduce an outside sexual partner into your relationship. It can confuse matters and stir up lots of other issues that will distract you from the work at hand. Taking a break from sex in your partnership can be a time to deepen your communication and trust. It can serve as a time to grow your relationship.

Once you have negotiated your time off from sex, set a date about halfway through to check in with each other. Also set a date at the end of the time out to talk and renegotiate, if needed. What have you gotten out of it? What have you learned? Are you ready to be sexual now? Do you want to be sexual? What will continue to move your healing forward?

> My boyfriend and I arranged to take a break from sex for three months, and then extended it to six months. It was really hard for me to ask for this. I didn't know if he'd love me still if we weren't having sex. We worked on our relationship a lot during this time, and I feel like it has made us stronger.—Hannah

Many survivors never negotiate a break from sex because they are afraid of their partner's response. They continue to have sex out of fear. But most partners respond positively to this request. They are glad to be proactive about sex and learn a lot themselves during this time. If your partner is unwilling to take a break, you can be thankful for such clarity. This is important information to know about your partner. You can consider whether you are compatible as partners through this healing process. You may not be. This can be very painful—but do you really want to be sexual with someone who cannot support you right now?

A break from partner sex can be a time to explore your sexuality on your own. Through masturbation, you can work with your triggers and establish a different relationship with your own body and sexuality. You may also want to take a break from sex with yourself. If so, follow the same model as when negotiating a break with a sexual partner. What do you want to accomplish during this time? What do you want to work on? How can you be intimate with yourself? If you take a break, be conscious about it. Set a date to check in with yourself about being sexual again.

When I took a break from having sex with other people, I really took charge of my own sexuality. I learned how to respect myself enough to say "no," and then I said "yes" to sex with myself. I learned about sex with my own timing and agenda.—Anita

This work asks you to be both gentle and courageous. See yourself as powerful and capable of healing sexually. Sexual healing can be hard and scary work at times, but the benefits of getting your body and sexuality back are profound.

Sex Guide Exercises

1. What triggers you? What acts, states of mind, or feelings can trigger you? Be specific. What happens in your body when you are triggered? What repeating images, sounds, or memories emerge when you are triggered?
2. What actions can you take proactively to work with your sexual triggers outside of a sexual setting?
3. Prepare a Trigger Plan on your own or with a partner. Share this with your partner, a friend, or a counselor. Add your own ideas to the Many Choices list for dealing with triggers.

chapter twelve

The Emotions of Healing:

You Gotta Feel Your Way Out of This

Once I let myself feel guilty, lonely, and angry during sex, I began to deal with all of the ways incest had affected my sexuality.—Carla

Many survivors are afraid to feel. You may be afraid that if you let yourself feel the depth of your loss, you will never stop crying. Or that if you let yourself feel the extent of your rage, you will hurt yourself or someone, else. But I have never seen anyone caught in an emotion forever—once they were willing to feel it. Usually the fear of the emotion is worse than actually feeling it.

Emotions are your travel buddies on the road to sexual healing. You can't heal if you can't feel. You certainly can't enjoy the pleasures of intimate sex if you cannot access all of your emotions.

Most of us survived the abuse by tuning out our emotions. Through dissociation, we escaped the emotions that were too unbearable to feel at the time. These unfelt emotions, or unprocessed trauma, are stored in our bodies, minds, and spirits, awaiting healing. Every survivor I've known has, at some point, wished this pain would magically disappear, but that doesn't seem to be how it works. Feeling and healing emotionally is the ticket out.

I thought that having sex meant that I was supposed to feel happy all the time and satisfied, but I often felt pissed off and lonely after sex. I figured I must be doing something wrong.—Cindy

You may think feeling bad means you aren't making progress in your healing. This is a mistake. We all hope that healing will feel good; but mostly, it doesn't. Healing can feel more like dying—dying and being transformed, and then finding yourself changed for the better, with a life of your own.

You Have to Feel It to Heal It

Emotions are our responses to life. As we move through our lives, we experience the richness of love and delight, the emptiness of loss, and the fire of dedication and anger. Emotions are felt as bodily sensations. Here is another area of healing in which embodiment pays off. As you become more aware of the sensations in your body, you will gain access to the subtleties and intricacies of your emotions.

You want to build an emotional flexibility that lets you move easily from one emotional state to another, from sadness to longing and desire, from irritation to joy and pleasure, and so on. Each new emotion helps you build your emotional range. The greater your range, the easier it will be for you to shift from one emo-

The Variety of Emotions and Moods

What is your emotional range? How do these emotions show up as sensations in your body?

enthusiasm

excitement

sadness

grief

joy

peace

ease

loss

anger

irritation

settledness

groundedness

confusion

anticipation

surprise

fear

terror

ambition

love

feeling loved

spiritual longing

sexiness

boredom

tion to the next. You will be less likely to feel stuck in an emotional rut, experiencing the same emotion, such as fear, over and over until it has a stranglehold on your life.

Emotions occur naturally and automatically, and they are designed for expression and healing. Unfelt or "held" emotions will remain in your system until they are acknowledged. If they are never attended to, they can run amok, affecting your physical, mental, and spiritual health. Unprocessed traumatic experiences and emotions color the lenses through which you view your reality. For instance, many adult survivors feel profoundly powerless long after they really are no longer powerless.

I see our emotions as self-healing mechanisms that help us maintain our mental and spiritual health. Grief and anger are natural responses to hurt and trauma, serving as healing agents to mend our wounds. When we are able to feel the depths of these emotions, we experience transformation and release. That metamorphosis and return to empowerment is what we mean by *healing*.

Chances are you've wondered how you can feel contradictory emotions, such as sadness and relief or anger and compassion, at the same time. I've worked with many survivors who insist, "My feelings don't make sense!" But emotions follow their own set of rules. Emotional logic and cognitive logic operate quite differently; our emotional systems are vast enough to hold contradictions that don't make sense to our way of thinking. You may feel both love and hate for your perpetrator—most survivors do. You may feel terrified of facing the feelings left over from your abuse, yet long to do so. These contradictions are natural to the logic of emotions. The trick is making room in our *minds* for the possibility of these contradictions.

The Five Stages of Emotions

Emotions and emotional expression follow a predictable cycle. The cycle of emotions can be like a wave building to fullness and crashing on the beach, then reintegrating into the ocean only to come to shore once more.

I've broken this process down into five stages:

First, the emotion shows up as a sensation or feeling. The emotion may be a response to either a current or a past experience. Of course, emotions from the past will emerge as you heal.

Then you have a choice. You can turn away from the emotion or you can open toward it. There are times when putting an emotion on hold is a good way of taking care of yourself. Holding emotions down doesn't work as a way of life, however. The longer you brace against emotions, particularly those wrought by abuse, the longer those emotions will run your life.

Instead of turning way from the emotions, you can choose to welcome them. In stage two of the cycle, you attend to the emotion, feeling your way *into* the sensation. When you do this, the emotion tends to intensify and reveal itself. This stage can often be the scariest. Just as in healing from dissociation, feeling your emotions means learning to tolerate these sensations in your body.

> ### *The Five Stages of Emotions*
>
> 1. Sensations and emotions emerge.
>
> 2. As you attend to or turn toward the emotions, they intensify and increase.
>
> 3. Emotions grow to a point of fullness, like water about to spill over the top of a bowl.
>
> 4. Emotions release or are expressed bodily.
>
> 5. Intentionally complete the cycle. Draw upon your internal emotional resources.

Stage three brings the emotion to fullness. The emotion grows in its charge and sensation. You may feel like you are about to cry. Your chest may overflow with joy and pleasure. You may want nothing more than to throw a major tantrum.

Stage four brings release. Depending upon the emotion, you may experience this release as gentle or very intense. You may sweat or blush, sob, shake, tremble, kick, laugh, yell, or become overheated or chilled. This expression is the release of the emotion. Surprisingly, the full expression of even the most intense and scary emotions usually lasts only twenty minutes at most.

After the full expression of the emotion, you may find relief, peace, renewed energy, and a sense of healing or transformation. This is the completion of the cycle, or what some people call *integration*. Take time to be with yourself. Breathe. Check in with your internal sense of safety and well-being (see chapter 1). Notice that you are alright, that you were not harmed in the process of healing. Acknowledge that you are complete with this piece of your healing; it can be helpful to say this out loud. Bring intentionality to this part of the process.

Orgasms follow this same cycle. Surprised?

Pay attention to the completion stage. Sometimes you may find yourself pouring out emotion with no experience of change or integration. You could be recycling the trauma rather than healing it. I do not encounter this often—most people who are not ready for healing try to repress emotions related to the abuse. But if this is happening to you, ask yourself, "What would it take to complete this feeling?" If you don't know the answer, make one up. Imagine you know what completion would feel like. Try it on for size.

Once you face, feel, release, and complete traumatic emotions, you will be free to build intimate, sexual relationships. Instead of being weighed down by the burden of your past, you'll need carry with you only enough faith and courage to meet the fears and risks love requires of us all.

Take a moment to consider which stages in the cycle of emotions you are good at and which you need to practice. Are you able to express your emotions, or do you tend to hold or repress them? Can you complete a cycle of emotion and move to integration? Where can you use more support or learning?

Emotional Centering

Sensations are the basis of emotions. Think about your favorite color or piece of music, or a place you where you experience peace or beauty. Notice what happens to your sensations. Your chest might relax and open, your belly settle, or your legs feel a pleasant streaming. How do you know when you are happy or upset? Where in your body do you feel that?

Noticing your emotions as sensations enables you to become emotionally flexible, moving more easily between emotional states and having room enough internally to both experience and interpret your emotions as they happen.

This is also what is meant by being *emotionally centered*. When you are emotionally centered, you are able to hang with your emotions, to notice them, feel them, and attend to them, yet not have them run you. Being emotionally centered allows you to fully experience your feelings and take care of yourself at the same time. With practice, you can learn how to have your emotions fully and make your own choices about them. Developing this kind of emotional center is a skill you will use in bringing intimacy and sex together. You will also use it in your sexual healing process.

We become accustomed to interpreting certain sensations as certain emotions. For example, the sensations of fear may feel similar to the sensations of excitement or titillation. The sensations of being grounded can feel much like those of boredom or being stuck. Be curious about your sensations. Are you feeling fear? Or are you opening up? Once you learn to differentiate sensations and emotions, subtlety comes into play.

> *I was fantasizing about sex with this guy I've been attracted to for a long time. I was masturbating, and I got to this edge I've reached before that feels like old fear about the abuse. Instead of checking out or trying to get away from it, I stayed with it. The most amazing thing happened. Upon closer examination, what felt like fear was sexual excitement. The feeling kind of opened up then and became very pleasant and alive.—Danielle*

Be careful when interpreting your emotions. It will not help you just to "re-interpret" terror as excitement when it really *is* terror. Gently releasing and feeling the terror will heal it for you.

Emotional Sourcing

Imagine that you had a deep internal well of emotional resources to dip into when the going gets tough. Facing your feelings might not seem so terrible if you knew the emotional support you needed was available right inside of you. Emotional sourcing helps you develop positive, pleasurable places in yourself from which to approach your healing.

To create emotional sourcing for yourself, bring your attention to any pleasant, peaceful, or settled sensation you can find in your body right now. Can you find a spot in your body where you feel warmth spreading? A sense of relaxation? If you can't find a source of pleasure in your body, try imagining an object that gives you pleasure—the beautiful shirt you are wearing, a seashell or stone you found, or a special gift from a dear friend. Maybe your source will be a place in nature. If you find yourself smiling, you've got it! Now let yourself enter those sensations. Notice where the feelings of pleasure show up in your body. Get to know them.

When you reach a difficult piece of your healing, a moment you think you just will not survive, you can go back to your emotional source. Use that internal source of support to center yourself and help you gain perspective on your recovery. This will ease the process of working through difficult emotions and traumas.

Emotional Healing

I am afraid that if I let myself start crying I will never stop. —Sheila

As you heal, you will likely work with anger, grief, a sense of betrayal, blaming yourself, and placing accountability on the offender, shame, terror, a sense of your own internal resources and courage, longing, and compassion and forgiveness for yourself. I have found that survivors who are willing to face these emotions develop both courage and calmness.

Anger and Rage

I am scared to death of my anger. I am afraid that if I express it, really let it out, it will take over my life. I will be some mad, raging woman, screaming at the world.—Chris

My anger has saved my life. My anger has been the juice that let me know I was worth something.—Daren

When it comes to expressing your anger and rage about having been sexually abused as a girl, there is only one rule:

Do not hurt yourself or anyone else, or break any object that is important to you or to anyone else.

Otherwise, you have free reign to let out all of that anger until you have expressed all that is useful to express.

Most survivors I have worked with are so concerned about *not* raging that it takes them a long time to learn to express any anger at all. You may be able to say, "I am angry," but *really* letting out the rage, expressing all the anger that you didn't get to express as a child, may be something else altogether.

Anger is energy you can use to protect yourself and to stand up for your rights and dignity. Now you can have the opportunity to benefit from your anger in the ways that you could not as a kid.

> *I found this amazing therapist a couple of years into my healing. She taught me to wail on huge pillows with a plastic bat. I felt like I was living a delayed reaction. Now I was getting to respond physically in all of the ways that weren't safe when I was a girl.—Stephanie*

For many survivors, anger emerges during sex. You may be angry that a memory or trigger is invading your sex life or pissed off at your own emotions, sensations, turn-on, or body. You may also feel angry at your partner. Suddenly, nothing your lover does is right and you can barely tolerate a touch that previously you may have delighted in. There's no mistaking this trigger. The past comes bubbling up and your hurt, fear, and anger get projected onto the closest target.

> *I find it much easier to get angry at my boyfriend, to harp on him about anything, than to direct my anger where it belongs. It is so much scarier to get angry at those who hurt me.—Debbie*

Well, it's time to get angry at those who hurt you. Go directly to the source. Get angry at the people who caused you this pain. Get mad at the people who failed to protect you. Express that anger in a way that works for you—scream at your pillow, lecture the wall, write a letter. Say everything you wanted to say long ago, but couldn't. Allow yourself to express what you have wanted all these years to express.

When you feel angry during sex, pause, breathe, and acknowledge that anger in some way. You may find it works for you to do this internally, or you may need to acknowledge the anger out loud. You may decide to acknowledge the anger in the moment or save it for your therapy group, a phone call to your best friend, or some other supportive setting. Feeling anger is a healthy part of being alive. Feeling intense anger is a *really* healthy response to being sexually abused as a child.

When feeling and expressing your anger, remember to breathe and to stay in your body. How does your body want to express this anger? You may feel silly, but let your body do what it wants to do. Many survivors were held down, trapped by the weight of their abusers, and terrorized or shamed into silence. You may want to push or hit, yell, curse, or kick. Any of these are fine, provided you do them safely.

Ways to Safely Express Your Anger

- Find a safe place where you can be loud and use your voice. Your bedroom, the shower, a secluded place in the woods, or your car are good choices. Make noise, growl, yell. Tell that abuser everything you have always wanted to say. Make noise as you...

- Physicalize your anger. Get a tennis racket or plastic bat and beat on pillows, your bed, or a couch. Breathe. Bend your knees so you don't injure your back.

- Twist a large towel in your hands, wringing your anger into it.

- Rip up old phone books. Tear them apart with your anger.

- Lie on a mattress or futon. Beat your fists and kick your legs on the surface. Push against something.

- Pile up cushions along the base of a couch, or stack cushions along a wall. Turn onto one side and kick in the pillows. If using a wall, ensure that there is enough padding, that you are safe, and that you do not break your toes or kick the wall in. Being able to kick your legs can be an amazing relief. Our legs and butts are the sites of the most powerful muscles in our bodies. We can move them with great force.

When you are ready, try expressing your anger with someone else present. This could be a close friend, another survivor, a support group, or your counselor or therapist. It can be difficult to learn to express your anger alone. Having someone witness your anger can be very powerful. When you are feeling small and vulnerable, it's great to have someone who can remind you of how you stood up for yourself.

Anger helps you reclaim your worthiness, dignity, and self-respect. Anger says, "No, this was not right. This is not acceptable!" You may feel relieved and peaceful after having expressed rage at what happened to you. I have seen many survivors develop confidence and compassion for themselves by learning to fully express anger.

Grief and Loss

> The question isn't have I ever cried during or after sex, but just how many times have I cried?—Stephanie

Under all that anger, you'll find loss and grief. We are angry because we have been disrespected, betrayed, and wounded—and we grieve for these same pains. For survivors, there is the loss of your body, your childhood, your love, your safety, and your fundamental ability to trust yourself, other people, the world, and in many cases, your mother, father, siblings, and other family members. Childhood sexual abuse is responsible for some of the most devastating losses that humans experience.

Grief and loss also come up during sex—including masturbation. Many survivors also report crying when they orgasm.

> For years I cried every time I had an orgasm. I thought it was strange and tried to stop it. Once I remembered being molested, it made sense.—Cheryl

> I can sob after I come. It feels like a big release of the grief of being incested and the relief of having my body and my life back.—Sally

Other survivors speak about a more generalized sense of loss during sex.

Having sex has this strange way of reminding me that I am an adult. I then get in touch with the childhood I never had. Where did it go? I have lots of grief there.—Pamela

Feeling sadness and grief while being sexual is a normal part of the healing process and can come up periodically throughout your life. Sex is about opening to all emotions that are present in us. A healthy sexual relationship can make room for your sadness, loss, and tears. Remember, the intensity of these feelings won't last forever. The more you allow yourself to feel and express an emotion, the sooner it will be done.

Grief can show up in many ways. You can shake, sweat, sob, moan, or laugh until you cry. Your chest may ache. You may want to curl up into a ball or crawl under the covers. Do what helps you feel deeply and release the loss from your insides. You may want to rock yourself, wrap yourself in a blanket and cry, or name aloud the things you have lost. You can make art about your loss and show it to others, or release it by burying it or burning it. Ritualizing loss can be powerful. You can make up a ritual that is meaningful to you to mark the official loss or grief and then let yourself mourn.

The Anger/Grief Interchange

Grief and anger can be mingled in a way that enables you to avoid one or the other. Most survivors I have worked with tend to favor either grief or anger. Those more comfortable with anger will go to anger automatically, even when they are feeling loss. Others, more comfortable with tears and sadness, will avoid feeling anger by crying. Or they will cry when they get mad.

Both anger and grief are vital to your health. Anger helps you learn to stand up for yourself, to draw the line as to what is acceptable and unacceptable to you. Anger vitalizes you. Loss and grief remind you that you are soft, human, and touchable. Loss demonstrates that you, too, have an effect on others. And to the extent that we can feel deep loss, we can also feel vast love and hold deep convictions. In this softness and vulnerability, we are also powerful.

Grief also allows us to move on. When we grieve, we feel deep sorrow and move through the process of letting go. It is in letting go that we can find change and completion. One day, you will remember the grief, loss, and abandonment of childhood sexual abuse and realize that those feelings have been completed for you. Grief no longer runs your heart, abandonment is no longer at the center of your fears, and loss no longer rules your life.

Do you lean toward anger or sadness? Which is the easier emotion for you? Try including the other emotion in your life. If you default to anger, ask yourself, *What is underneath my anger? What loss am I angry about?* We are usually angry about how we were hurt or what we have lost. If you default to tears and sadness, ask yourself, *Where is my anger? How can I begin to stand up for myself? What would it be like to be angry?*

Fear

Childhood sexual abuse is dangerous. When you were being abused, you may have felt like you were fighting to stay alive. Whether the struggle to survive was literal or metaphorical, fear, terror, and the real or perceived threat of death were visceral experiences for most survivors. This fear and terror can stay with you for years. Your body can get caught in a flight, fight, or freeze response, not knowing, on some level, that the abuse is long over.

This terror can show up during sex. You may find yourself feeling fear that doesn't seem to have anything to do with what is currently happening. You may be afraid to masturbate or afraid of sex altogether. A wave of terror may come over you in the midst of being sexual.

> *Sometimes I just get scared. There is no memory or trigger that I can tell...I just feel terrified. Sometimes I wonder if I'm still letting out all of the terror I froze inside me.*—Rosa

Fear is particularly tricky when you are being intimate with a lover. You can project past abuse and reactions onto your current sexual partner. This is all a natural part of healing, yet it can be challenging for your sexual relationships. During sex, your partner may remind you of one of your abusers. You may think he or she wants to betray you—just like your abusers did.

My boyfriend seems just like my dad sometimes when we are having sex. I become young and scared and he seems so big. I am convinced he wants to take something from me.—Jenifer

When feeling terror, you may shake or tremble, cough or sweat. You may freeze up and be unable to speak. These are normal responses to terror and probably similar to what you experienced as a child. See whether the fear is grounded in the present day or if it is a reaction to past abuse. What is happening in your life? Is there anything dangerous in your current situation you need to change?

If you are experiencing past fear emerging in your body, use your trigger plan to help you out. Stop, breathe, feel your body, get up and move around. Often, comforting yourself can be enough. Remind yourself that you are safe today, that the past *was* really scary, but that you are okay now. Call forth your internal sense of safety and access your emotional source. Physicalize your terror, allowing your body to move through the sensations.

I am absolutely committed to sitting in my own fear. I say, "I am afraid, I am so afraid, and I am going there anyway." Every time I do, some profound healing happens.—Akaya

Longing

Usually tucked amid the fear and grief is longing. You can long for what you wish you had or long for those aspects of your relationship with your abuser that you miss. Like many survivors, you might long for your mother or someone else who can protect you. You may yearn for a childhood in which you felt loved and safe.

My dad took me out camping and on outdoor adventures. I felt strong and like I could do anything. I also felt safe with him in these settings, protected. These are the experiences I miss.—Carla

Acknowledge your longing. While grief and anger at what was missing often comes with this, longing tells you what you need and what is important to you. If you are longing for love, you can go about bringing more love into your life. If you long for a sense of belonging or being known, you can take steps to create these experiences.

Longing often includes contradictions which may make you reluctant to acknowledge your longing. "How can I long for the person who hurt me the most in my life?" You may love the person who sexually abused you. In addition to being a perpetrator, that person was your father, brother, aunt, grandfather, or teacher. As uncomfortable as it may be, let yourself feel your longing. Longing opens your heart, and opening your heart is good for you. It is what will serve your life now.

I love my father still after all he did to me. I realize that if I pretend that I don't love him, I am closing off a piece of my heart. If I close off that place in my heart, nothing can get in there.—Danielle

Shame and Guilt

I have never met a survivor who did not believe, on some level, that the sexual abuse was her fault. I have never met a survivor who did not carry the shame and guilt of this.

The sexual abuse was not your fault. I could say this five times or five hundred times, and I would not have said it enough. The sexual abuse was not your fault. Even if you literally asked your abuser to touch you, the abuse was not your fault. The older or more powerful person was responsible for your care and well-being. Sexual abuse does not accomplish this.

Really getting it that the abuse was not my fault took a very long time. I had to be ready to feel how truly helpless and powerless I was at the time of the abuse. That I was vulnerable and dependent, and that I couldn't stop it.—Kassie

Shame lives very deeply for survivors. Somehow it is easier to believe that you are at fault than to feel the utter helplessness of having been abused. It may seem unimaginable that someone you love would hurt you on purpose. "It must be my fault," you think, "or why else would they do that?"

Survivors have many different reasons for feeling that their shame and guilt is deserved. However, there are some common themes: Many survivors believe the abuse was their fault because they didn't fight back, or because they had an orgasm during the abuse, or because they initiated an episode of the abuse, or because they should have been smart or resourceful enough to stop it. Other survivors feel marked or dirty, ashamed to have been the chosen victim.

Some survivors abused other kids as a way of acting out what was happening to them. This carries an immense load of guilt and shame. While you do not have to punish yourself, you can take responsibility for your actions. Depending upon your situation, you may want to make amends, if that will support your healing and that of the other person.

Some children are forced to abuse other kids, as is often the case in ritual abuse. If you had your choice of playing with friends in the backyard, going to get ice cream, or sexually abusing another kid, which would you have chosen? Playing in the yard or getting ice cream. Kids are manipulated into abusing others. While you are accountable for your actions as an adult, children sexually abusing other children is a situation created by adults.

You may also feel shame about experiencing pleasure or liking sex. Many survivors do. If you like sex, then you must have liked the abuse, right? No way! Experiencing sexual pleasure is your birthright. Sexual pleasure is fine, good, and acceptable.

Remedy your shame and guilt with regular megadoses of self-forgiveness and self-dignity.

Being Witnessed in Your Emotions

Being witnessed in the midst of your emotions is a powerful experience. Being witnessed means just having someone present with you as you feel your feelings. Your friend, lover, or support does not need to change or fix your feelings. She or he can simply witness witness. You can learn from others' acceptance of your emotions that you are truly okay. In my survivors' workshops, I notice that other survivors are relieved and happy when someone finally expresses anger, grief, or longing. Everyone seems to breathe a big sigh of relief.

You can ask for specific support from your witness or support person. You may want to be held or to rant and rave uninterrupted for twenty minutes. You can ask your support person take care of his or her own needs and boundaries. If the experience gets too intense, he or she can take a break.

Some people are comfortable with certain emotions and not with others. Your friend may be fine holding you when you cry, but freak out when you get really angry. Your emotions are not "too much" or "too intense." Expressing any degree of anger, loss, or shame *in a safe way* is just fine. Your partner may simply not have developed the capacity to hang with that depth of emotion. Let your partner take care of his or her needs and limitations. Find a support person who can go with you where you need to go.

> My partner has learned over time. My rage used to scare him; now he is right with me as I kick the bed as hard as I can, yelling at my dad to get away from me.—Jeanie

You may find yourself wanting to ask for reassurance. Go ahead and ask. Look at your partner. Let yourself see that someone is there. Ask, "Do you think this is bad?" "Am I hurting you?" "How is this for you?" You may need a reality check as you are learning to express this depth of emotion.

Sex Guide Exercises

1. Practice your emotional centering and sourcing. How does this practice change how you move through your triggers and sexual healing?
2. Choose three different emotions connected to your sexual healing (for example, guilt, anger, and grief). One by one, write about the following for each emotion:
   a. What body sensations let me know that I am feeling this emotion?
   b. What is it like to be in my body and feel my sensations while having this emotion? How much tolerance do I have for this emotion?
   c. Review "The Five Stages of Emotions" in this chapter. Do you tend to get stuck in any particular stage? Is this different for different emotions?
   d. How can I feel and express this emotion? How can I practice completing it?

chapter thirteen

S/M, Role-Playing, and Fantasy

Sex is complex. Your desires may not be tidy or fit into a design that is reflected in the mainstream version of sex. For most people, and particularly for survivors, sex is full of contradictions. Sex can be calm, aggressive, nurturing, and challenging—all at the same time. S/M, role-playing, and fantasies are tools you can use to explore and express sexuality.

S/M 101: Consent, Power, Sensation

S/M is short for *sadomasochism*, a term that has been used by the psychological establishment to label sadistic and masochistic behaviors. People who practice S/M, however, use this term as one of identification and empowerment. S/M refers to a sexual preference that can include power play, intense sensations, pain, bondage, and role-playing.

Most people associate S/M with images of black leather, bondage, spanking, and whipping. In the early 1990s, Madonna's photo book *Sex* made S/M chic. Since then, mainstream culture has adopted S/M imagery, exposing the general public to S/M as a sexual practice.

For S/M practitioners, including survivors of childhood sexual abuse, S/M can be a powerful, sensate arena for sexual exploration. Many practitioners talk about the safety of S/M, the power of negotiating sexual play, and the potential for sexual healing and self-empowerment through S/M.

The ground rules of S/M are the basically same as in vanilla sex (the term used by S/M practitioners for non-S/M sex). S/M is practiced between two or more consenting adults. The S/M community is very outspoken about consent. Before engaging in S/M play, the partners discuss their desires, interests, and limits to create a scene in which they can play erotically and safely. Negotiable items include who will participate, what will happen, where, when, and how. Who will be the top? Who the bottom? If you think of S/M as a willing exchange of power between consenting adults, the top is the person who is wielding power and directing the action. The bottom is surrendering power to the top within carefully negotiated parameters. Partners agree upon a "safeword," which is a code word used to call all activity to a halt, if so desired. Genital contact and orgasm may or may not be a part of an S/M scene.

A scene may include fantasy roles or characters, bondage, pain, and/or power play. Some players construct elaborate fantasies, with fully costumed characters. Maid and master, older woman and young man, nurse and patient, cop and motorist are common roles people play with. It's the strong power differential that sets up the dynamic. You can construct an S/M scene from any dynamic that turns you on. S/M play often involves bondage, blindfolding or other sensory control, and restrictions on movement, behavior, and speech. Sensation play can include whipping with soft deerskin floggers, over-the-knee spankings, caning and paddling, nipple play with clamps or clothespins, and playing with hot wax— to name a few.

S/M players tend to speak about intensity of sensation, rather than pain *per se*. As you become sexually aroused—whether in S/M or vanilla play—endorphins are released in the body, creating chemical changes. Your threshold for stimulation and pain increases with the production of endorphins. S/M plays with this phenomenon in a way that many people find enjoyable. What looks like it would hurt (and well might when you are not turned on) might be very pleasurable in the right context!

Exploring the Edges

Some people will tell you S/M is abusive, perverted, or wrong—in short, a "bad" way to express your eroticism. Many of the arguments against people who eroticize power play are the same ones that are used against gays, lesbians, and bisexuals. And these same arguments have been used against women who have wanted to empower themselves sexually, and against sex itself.

If you enjoy topping, bottoming, power play, or other S/M eroticism, you are not alone. Many survivors find power play very erotic. Exploring the edges of your own limits and challenging your partners to find theirs can have its place in an empowered sex life.

The hottest sex I have is in S/M scenes. The taboo of our scenes and the places I get to find in myself are amazing. I get to surrender as a bottom in a way I have never surrendered.—Rey

S/M is important to me. I don't want any more violence connected to sex, or any more people hurting kids or adults sexually. S/M is not that. I am turned on by power play, bondage, and whipping. These are very deep and intimate experiences with my partner. It is not about hurting either one of us...rather it is about expressing a very deep part of myself.—Kassie

Many survivors play with shame, control, and punishment. This is a hot button for many of us; after all, shame and punishment were means of controlling us as children. You can construct a scene in which a top "threatens" a bottom with punishment for "misbehavior." In the S/M community, this is called "emotional edge play."

Being an S/M top is finally where I feel at home. I was reluctant to get into S/M. I was afraid that I would hurt someone or take out my rage in the wrong place. The opposite seems to be true. I feel closer to my partners, more caring, and I feel more myself.—Melanie

Enacting rape scenes in which you can be "taken" in some way is a popular S/M fantasy. Here you can play with the dynamic of being sexually overwhelmed (or taking control of your partner) in a consensual and safe context.

> *Rape scenes are very exciting for me. As I say "no," my partner teases me and talks about how much I want it. This is cathartic and makes all of the abuse stuff less threatening. It gives me more of a sense of control.*—Jenifer

S/M and Survivors

The impact of childhood sexual abuse shows up in S/M play just as in any other kind of sex play. Some survivors who are into S/M consciously work with their history of abuse in their scenes. This can be done in a number of ways. You can explore sexual acts and positions in which you were abused. You may find it powerful to reenact abuse scenes and write new endings for them. By reentering the scenario in a safe place with a safe person, you can change your experience of the abuse.

> *I reenacted abuse scenes in S/M. This freaks some survivors out, but I got so much power back out of it. I cried and worked through the way the abuse had turned me on. I also saw how powerful I am now in comparison to how small I was then. It brought me compassion for myself and a sense that he could never get me again.*—Rebecca

Some S/M players explore age play, taking on teacher/student or other age-differentiated roles. Others combine age play with gender play; these are specific constructs which have a long history in the S/M community. These roles provide a context to play with the dynamics of nurturing, mentoring, control, and dependence.

This can be very intense for survivors. If you are going to engage in role-playing that in any way resembles your abuse, prepare yourself and your partner well for it. Make sure your partner is aware of the possible emotional triggers or release that this kind of scene may evoke for you. Be sure to choose a safeword that you will remember if triggered. I suggest that you and your partner establish a good foundation of trust before you engage in this type of scene.

While you'll learn a lot about yourself, this type of S/M play is not a substitute for therapy or any other type of concentrated healing from your abuse. Some survivors use S/M as a tool to explore the impact of abuse in a very direct manner. Just as with survivors who prefer vanilla sex, survivors who like S/M find that their sex lives get better and their scenes more satisfying as they are embodied and healing from their abuse.

S/M as "Acting Out" Abuse

Within communities of abuse survivors, S/M is a controversial sexual practice and tends to stir up a lot of debate. Almost everyone has an opinion about S/M. Because it is a marginalized sexual practice, many people are uniformed about how S/M really works. They are concerned about combining sex with what looks like violence.

The most often debated question is whether S/M players are "acting out" prior abuse. My answer is both yes and no, depending. I have interviewed a number of survivors who practice S/M and have done somatic work with many more. At Good Vibrations, I talked with hundreds of customers about their S/M practices. I found that survivors can and do use S/M as a way to dissociate and to unsuccessfully process the abuse. Of course, survivors check out during vanilla sex, too, and use vanilla sex as a way to escape feelings. You can try to complete an unfinished trauma by unconsciously replaying it over and over again, in S/M or any other kind of sex.

> *I struggled in the S/M community. I did things that were extreme because I was used to extremes in sex. It was all I knew. I didn't know how to be in my body enough to have boundaries. I was used to having things done to me.—Marty*

> *There is a difference between surrender and abdication. I am not abdicating any of my capacity to make decisions for myself, but I am choosing to surrender.—Aurora*

Sexual energy in and of itself is neutral. You can have sex in a way that is creative and healing for you, or in a way that keeps you disembodied and at risk.

What is particularly intense for those observing S/M from the outside is seeing sexuality combined with something that looks much like violence. Sexual violence is all around us. We hear disturbing reports of molested children, battered and murdered women, and rape as a war tactic. Thankfully, many of us are working to end sexual violence. S/M, however, is *not* sexual violence. First, S/M is consensual sexual play between adults. Second, S/M practitioners negotiate their scenes as equal partners. Third, S/M players employ safewords to stop the play immediately when necessary. Choice and control remain intact in the S/M experience. The bottom is not *really* out of control, and the scene may look more intense from the outside than it actually is. Violence allows for neither choice nor control.

S/M *does* explore an edge of human sexual expression. In every practice, from business to therapy, there are folks who dare to play on the margins, taking risks, and exploring what new experiences may have to offer. Innovation usually happens in the margins and then makes its way to the mainstream. No matter what your position on S/M, what we can appreciate about edgy practices is that they challenge us to take our imaginations further out than what might make us comfortable.

Survivors have all kinds of experiences in S/M play. Some survivors may feel they are "acting out" abuse, and others praise S/M for being an arena in which they can heal their abuse and fully claim their sexuality.

Some people in the S/M community argue that power dynamics are at play in all sexual relationships. S/M makes these dynamics overt and agreed upon, instead of covert and nonconsensual.

If a survivor ever tells me that she doesn't have to deal with power and its relation to sex in her life, I think she's lying.—Jenifer

Expressing your eroticism in a way that builds your self-esteem, helps you become more embodied, and encourages you have more pleasure in your life is the crux of any sexual choice.

Whether you are attracted to S/M or upset by the idea, you can educate your-self further by reading books written by S/M practitioners. You'll find lots of resources in the back of the book.

Vanilla Role-Playing

Folks who do not practice S/M may still like to play erotically with roles and characters. The variety of characters is limited only by your imagination. You'll probably find that certain dynamics and characters stay with you over time. You may want to play with gender or sexual orientation. You can let a part of you out that you normally do not express fully. You can be a movie star, a vamp, a god-dess, or a dominatrix. Role-playing can open up your possibilities, letting you become a lot more flexible in your sexual expression.

> *My lover and I like to dress up. He'll actually dress as the woman and I as the man. We trade and intensify the gender roles. It is a great turn-on and very intimate because we are both stretching our comfort zones.—Halli*

Fantasy

Fantasies are fertile ground for exploring your desires. Here's a way to heat up your sex life. You can use your imagination to try out a new sexual idea before you enact it. You can delight in new lovers, make love in risky places, or take on a new sexual role—all in the privacy of your own mind. The more flexible your thinking and fantasizing about sex, the better your sex life will be.

> *One of my favorite things to do is to tell my lover a fantasy while we are mak-ing love. It is yummy. I put us both into the fantasy, talking us through hot sex scenes and erotic terrain. Sometimes I'll make him a prince from a neighboring kingdom and me the princess heir to the throne. One time I turned him into a frog. That made us laugh.—Jeanie*

I have found that survivors often feel ashamed about fantasies that involve force, rape, incest, or sexual aggression of any kind. Somehow we got the idea that our fantasies are supposed to be filled with flowers and soft music. Lots of survivors fantasize about rape and other scenarios that include some form of power exchange. Some rape fantasies are violent, others romanticized. Some survivors get years of pleasure from these fantasies, while others are disturbed by them.

No fantasy is inherently "bad." There are no "right" or "wrong" fantasies. Instead of labeling your fantasy, consider whether it affects you positively or negatively.

I have only two concerns about fantasies. First, do you check out when you have the fantasy? Don't use fantasies to avoid being present with yourself or your partner. You don't want to practice being disembodied or dissociated when you are sexual. In fact, rather than a way to get out of a sexual encounter, fantasies can be a different way to be present and embodied. Being embodied can make your fantasy life all the richer.

My second concern is that you have more than one fantasy in your repertoire. Do you have only one fantasy? Is that fantasy the only way you can get off? Although such a fantasy often will closely resemble the dynamics of the abuse, the content is of less concern to me than the fact of being stuck in one fantasy that is replayed over and over. Part of healing is allowing more flexibility in your thinking and more freedom in your choices. Treat an intrusive fantasy that disturbs you as you would a trigger. Use the tools in chapter 11 for help.

Of course, survivors do use fantasies to work through abuse dynamics and memories. I have found that survivors are amazingly creative with this type of sexual fantasy.

> ### *Invent a Fantasy*
>
> Invent a fantasy right now. Go with whatever comes to mind that feels erotic to you. Where does your fantasy take place? What is the environment like? Who are the characters in your fantasy? Notice the sensations in your body as your story unfolds. What are you doing? What is the buildup? What kind of sex do you have? What about this fantasy turns you on?

I have this long-standing jail fantasy. There is a man behind bars and I go up to the bars and make him suck my dick. (I don't have a dick in real life, but in my fantasies I do.) He likes it, but I have the control. I don't let him stop until I want him to. I get off and leave him there. I think this fantasy has helped me get a lot of my power back from my brother and his abuse.—Marie

Sex Guide Exercises

1. What would you like to learn about S/M, role-playing, and fantasies?
2. If you are interested in S/M, brainstorm a list of activities, roles, or scenes you would be interested in.
3. If you are interested in role-playing, create a list of characters you would find erotic or intriguing to play with.

chapter fourteen

Sex Toys and Accoutrements

There are lots of ways to play sexually and lots of toys to play with. Sex toys can add a new dimension to your sex life. Sex toys can allow you to be in more places at once, or even add anatomy that you do not normally have! Many women prefer to orgasm with vibrators, too.

> *The first time I put on a dildo and harness I found it so empowering. It was like "Look! I have this and both hands!" I also got that guys must feel vulnerable walking around with their genitals hanging on the outside.—Stephanie*

You may have gotten the idea that sex toys are weird or perverted. Who knew that they have been used cross-culturally for centuries? Sex toys offer just another set of possibilities for your sexual pleasure.

Until recently, you most likely bought your sex toys at a porn shop or adult novelty store that catered primarily to men. While some folks like the explicitly sexual aura of these stores, others find the atmosphere very uncomfortable. Some men patronizing these shops can be surprised to see women shopping there.

Luckily, more women-run sex stores are opening in the United States, Canada, and Europe. Most of these stores offer sex-positive sex information right alongside quality toys and books on sex. You can find supportive, sex-positive sex toy stores in London, New York, Boston, Northampton, Toronto, Madison, Austin,

San Francisco, Berkeley, Seattle, Vancouver and other cities. I have listed a number of these shops in the Resources section, as well as mail-order companies. You do not have to live in a large urban center to have access to quality sex toys and information.

Truly, this is a great time to be interested in sex toys. More quality toys are available, many of them designed and produced by women. Vixen Creations, a woman-owned company based in San Francisco, has become one of the largest producers of high-quality silicone dildos and butt plugs. Stormy Leather, another woman-owned company in San Francisco, specializes in leather dildo harnesses, erotic clothing, and S/M paraphernalia. Of course, Good Vibrations, the original "clean well-lighted place to buy sex toys," is still serving men and women with great success in San Francisco, Berkeley, and Brookline, MA, as well as on the Web.

Vibrators

Vibrators were initially used by the medical profession to cure "female troubles," also called "hysteria" and considered to be a disturbance of the womb. Doctors used the vibrator to assist in medical massages aimed at causing "hysterical paroxysm" or orgasm in women. *Hmmmmm.*

The late 1800s produced a steam power massager, and by the early 1900s, numerous vibrating massagers were available to physicians along with textbooks on vibratory massage techniques. By this time, vibrators were seen as a cure for numerous ailments in both men and women. Until the end of the 1920s, vibrators could be purchased as home appliances for pleasure and health. The use of the massager for medical purposes declined with its appearance in porn films in the late 1920s. From then until the 1970s, vibrators were not advertised for their sexual uses. Many are still sold as back massagers, with no reference to their erotic uses.

Battery-Operated and Electric Vibrators

You can choose from electric and battery-operated vibrators. Battery-operated vibrators tend to be smaller and shaped like a long cucumber. The vibration of battery-operated devices tend to be weaker, and the quality of the products is not quite as reliable. They're great when you do not have an electrical outlet handy. Battery-operated vibrators will last anywhere from one to nine months, depending upon use.

Electric vibrators, on the other hand, are higher-quality devices and can last for years. There are two types of electric or plug-in vibrators: coil operated and motor driven. Coil-operated vibrators tend to be smaller and a bit quieter, with a

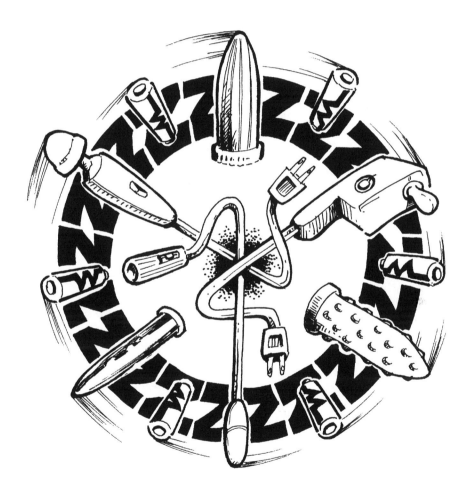

ILLUSTRATION 5. Vibrators

subtler vibration than that of the motor-run models. Motor-run vibrators are good for folks who like more stimulation. The vibration is stronger and the device a bit larger.

Some folks complain that the cord gets in the way when using an electric vibrator. If you invest in an electric vibrator, buy an extension cord as well. This gives you more room for movement, and you do not have to have sex right next to the wall socket.

There are now rechargeable electric vibrators. Depending on the model, these vibrators will hold their charge from thirty minutes to a few hours. You then need to plug them in again for two to six hours to recharge them.

You may recognize some of the brand names of vibrators from your kitchen appliances. Oster, Sunbeam, and Hitachi make high-quality vibrators. They are packaged as massagers and can be found in higher-quality sex stores as well as general department stores.

Vibrator Attachments

Various attachments are available for electric vibrators. They are generally soft and pliable and fit over the head of the motor-driven vibrators and on the attachment stem of coil-operated vibrators. Some of the attachments are designed to focus the vibration on a smaller spot (the clittickler), for penetration (the G-spotter), or for stimulating the head of the penis (the come cup). The attachments can add versatility to the toy.

A few opinions about these attachments: The nerves within the vaginal passage respond more to movement and pressure than to vibration. While some women like to use vibrators vaginally, do not be disappointed if this is not a big "wow" for you. If you use a vibrator vaginally, keep in mind that the lower third of the vagina tends to be the most responsive to vibration. Also, quite a bit of pressure is needed to stimulate the G-spot, and most attachments are too soft for G-spot stimulation.

Your anus is well suited to enjoying vibration. But if you are using an attachment for anal stimulation, make sure it has a flanged base. That is, the base must be wider than the end being inserted; this prevents the toy from accidentally slipping into the anal canal. Unlike the vagina, which is a closed system, the anal canal leads directly into the large intestine and into your body. A better bet for anal vibration is to insert a dildo, butt plug, or fingers into the rectum and press a vibrator into the base of the toy or the palm of your hand. The vibration will then be transmitted through the toy or your hand.

Dildos and Harnesses

Dildos are sex toys designed for penetration and are used by both men and women for sexual pleasure. You can use them vaginally or anally or both. Most dildos are made of silicone or plastic materials, and they come in various sizes and shapes, including penises, goddess figurines, dolphins, and nondescript shapes of various lengths and thicknesses.

Silicone dildos are of much higher quality than their plastic counterparts. Silicone is a nonporous material, so dirt and bacteria cannot work their way into your dildo. You can sterilize silicone dildos by boiling them for up to five minutes. Silicone is easy to warm before use by placing it in a hot bowl of water or running it under warm tap water. It will also absorb your body's heat with use. Silicone tends to have a smoother texture and to slide more easily, although you will still need to use a water-based lubricant, as with all dildos. As long as you keep sharp objects away from your silicone dildo (including the teeth and claws of curious dogs and cats!), it will last a long time. If the seal of the surface is cut or broken, silicone will crumble.

The benefits of plastic dildos lie primarily in price; for the most part, they are less expensive than silicone. Plastic dildos also tend to be available in larger models, for you size queens! The plastic materials are porous and can get dirty quickly. I recommend using condoms over plastic dildos even when using them with yourself. You'll have a much better chance of keeping them clean longer. Plastic dildos come in various textures and looks; the most "realistic" styles, those resembling a penis with balls, are made of this material.

So, why use dildos? Some women like the feel of a dildo better than a hand or penis. Some use dildos so they can be filled up both anally and vaginally at the same time. Dildos can be used when masturbating or when your partner is tired. You can pick the dildo of the exact size that fits you, which you can't do with your partner's hand or penis. You may want to be penetrated with something much larger (or smaller) than what nature can provide. Finally, with a dildo, you, too, can be endowed with the anatomy to penetrate your partners, whether you are sexual with men or with women.

Dildos can be used by hand or secured with a harness. Most harnesses are designed to wear around your hips, through a newer thigh harness is growing in popularity. Most harnesses are made of leather which tends to be soft on the skin, secure, and durable. Harnesses are also available in a neoprene and webbing design, for folks who do not like leather. These are less expensive, too.

The two main hip harness designs are distinguished by the number of straps holding them to your body. One style has a center strap that runs between your legs, like a G-string. This model can give the harness wearer clitoral stimulation. The second style

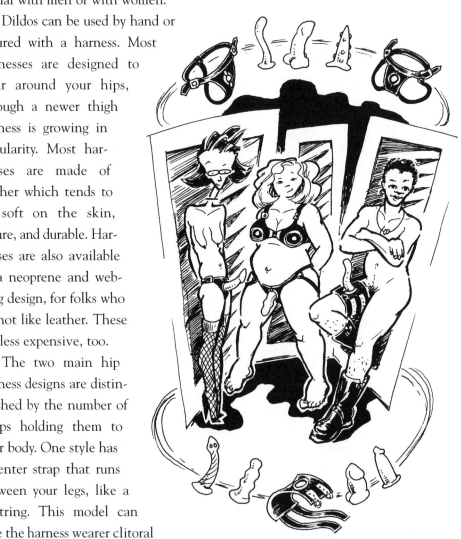

ILLUSTRATION 6. Dildos and Harnesses

has two straps that ride around the outside of each buttock and hip, like a jock-strap. These harnesses provide easier access to the genitals of the wearer.

Certain harnesses accommodate dildos with balls better than others. These have two straps that slide freely around the center ring used to secure the dildo, allowing you to arrange the straps around the balls on the dildo. This style of harness best accommodates men, allowing room for the penis to be tucked to the side comfortably. A man may strap one on if he has an erectile dysfunction, if he wants to keep playing after having come, if his partner wants to go longer than he can last, or for variety in width and length.

Harnesses with a piece of leather or cloth behind the base of the dildo are more comfortable for the harness wearer. The dildo does not end up pulling on your pubic hairs.

There are also thigh harnesses that you strap around your leg. Most often these are made of leather with wide bands of Velcro used to secure the harness. Thigh harnesses gives you new variety in positions and let you use the strength of your leg in penetration instead of your hips. You and your partner can each wear a thigh harness for simultaneous penetration. They can be used for vaginal and anal penetration.

Anal Toys

There are two rules when using toys for anal play; use lubrication and select a toy with a wide flanged base that will prevent it from sliding up inside of you or your partner.

Anal toys come in all shapes and sizes and in a variety of materials. There are butt plugs, dildos, anal vibrators, and anal beads. Butt plugs are wide in the middle and thinner at the end (of course, the base is wide enough to prevent the plug from slipping in). The idea is that the sphincter muscles can close around the plug, securing it in place. You can leave a plug in as you enjoy a variety of sexual activities. Placing a vibrator on the base of a butt plug can transmit vibrations into your rectum. This can feel great for many folks. Butt plugs are not designed for thrusting in and out of the anus; dildos are better for that.

Dildos are great for anal penetration. The idea is to choose the length and width that will be most enjoyable for you. Unlike a butt plug, a dildo will not stay secured in the anus without pressure. Dildos can be used by hand or with a harness. If you have not played much anally, start small so that you can experiment and learn how to relax your sphincter muscles. A good way to judge the desired width of an anal toy is to see how many fingers feel comfortable for you and use that as your guide.

Vibrators that are designed for anal use stimulate the very sensitive nerve endings in the anus. They can vibrate or twist and turn. Make sure you choose a quality toy for anal vibration, with plenty of material covering the internal moving parts. Some toys marketed for anal play are too shoddy to use safely.

Anal beads are pretty much what they sound like: a string of beads with a round hook or handle of some kind on one end. The beads are made of hard plastic or silicone, and come in a variety of sizes. Cheaper ones may have rough edges; use a nail file to smooth down any roughness that may injure your anal tissues. Many women and men sing the praises of anal beads, inserting them one at a time and then pulling them out during orgasm.

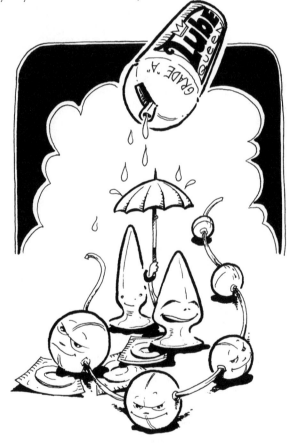

ILLUSTRATION 7. Anal Toys

Lubricants

Use a water-based lubricant with all of your toys. Lubricants will make sex play with dildos more pleasurable, and with anal toys they are a must. Some people prefer oil-based lubricants for anal play, because they don't evaporate with use. Remember that oils break down latex, so you should not use oil-based lubricants with latex condoms or gloves. Also, avoid getting oils in or near the vagina. Oils are hard for the natural cleansing mechanisms of the vagina to break down and may cause an infection. You can rehydrate water-based lubricants by adding water as you play. Placing some water or a spritzer bottle near your play space makes this easy.

> Lubricants saved my sex life. I thought I was damaged and broken because I never got very wet. I guess I just don't make a lot of juice. Lube is easy and works, and I don't feel like I am flawed.—Daren

Love Potions

There are lots of love potions on the market. Some claim they will enhance your sexual prowess, others that they will make you "last" longer. Mostly these are marketing strategies to interest you in the product. The biggest distinction is between those love potions that are edible and those that are not. The edible love potions will say so on the label; they are intended to be rubbed onto your partner's body and then licked or eaten off. You'll find hot and spicy flavors, fruit treats, and tubs of chocolate potions. Those that include more natural ingredients (i.e., have ingredients with words you can recognize) tend to be the most flavorful.

A number of love potions are made to cause sensations: they may be hot to the skin or heat up with rubbing. Kama Sutra makes a balm that has a slight, short-term numbing effect. This can be useful for people with very sensitive nipples.

You can make your own potions by adding scents and flavors to massage oil. You can play with edible spreads—from fruits to chocolate, from whipped cream to honey.

S/M and Bondage Toys

S/M and bondage toys include body harnesses, restraints, whips, canes, blind-folds, gags, collars, and erotic clothing—to name but a few. Much S/M and bondage gear is made of leather, latex, or PVC, which is a shiny vinyl. Some folks like to dress up in S/M fetish gear, even though they are not S/M practitioners.

If you are interested in this type of sexual expression, educate yourself. Because S/M can involve physical intensity and pain, it is important that you be skilled in what you are doing with S/M toys. Whips, ropes, and other toys can do harm in the hands of an uninformed player. *It is up to you to learn how to play safely.* Most S/M organizations offer workshops on basic safety, and books like *The New Bottoming Book* and *The New Topping Book* offer friendly instruction. See the Resources for more information.

When selecting S/M gear, be aware of the intensity of sensation your new toy will produce. If you are interested in nipple clamps, for example, the tweezer and alligator clips are adjustable and will give you some control over the intensity of the sensation. The tweezer style accommodates larger nipples. Marquis d'Clips and clothespins are nonadjustable; they provide much more intense sensation. The most intense sensation comes when the nipple clamps are removed.

Let's use whips as another example. There are various styles of whips with different names, made of leather, deer skin, rubber, and other materials, each creating a different sensation. Floggers are shorter whips made of many strands. Often they are crafted from fine leathers and feature thick, weighty strands. Most floggers create a heavy, deep sensation, while a long, thin whip will create a stinging sensation. A suede whip will give more of a thud that spreads sensation at first; it will give more sting as it collects body oils. A whip made of plastic will sting no matter what.

When learning how to use whips and other percussive S/M toys, practice on a pillow before you play with a partner. Learn how to aim the toy and how to produce the sensations you want. *It is essential that you learn how to wield your new toy safely.* Aim for the fleshy and muscled parts of the body—like the buttocks and upper back—and *always* steer clear of bones and internal organs.

Many folks play with bondage, whether or not they are into S/M. If you want to tie up your partner, you'll probably start by looking at household items. Some of the accoutrements you might find at home are dangerous choices for toys, however. Silk scarves and nylons are poor bondage devices because they can tighten when pulled, cutting off circulation or damaging the tissues. Bondage devices should be sturdy and comfortable to the wearer and not tighten with pressure and pulling. Your best bets are cloth or leather restraints made for the purpose. Remember to keep a pair of scissors near the bed for cutting off any bondage gone awry.

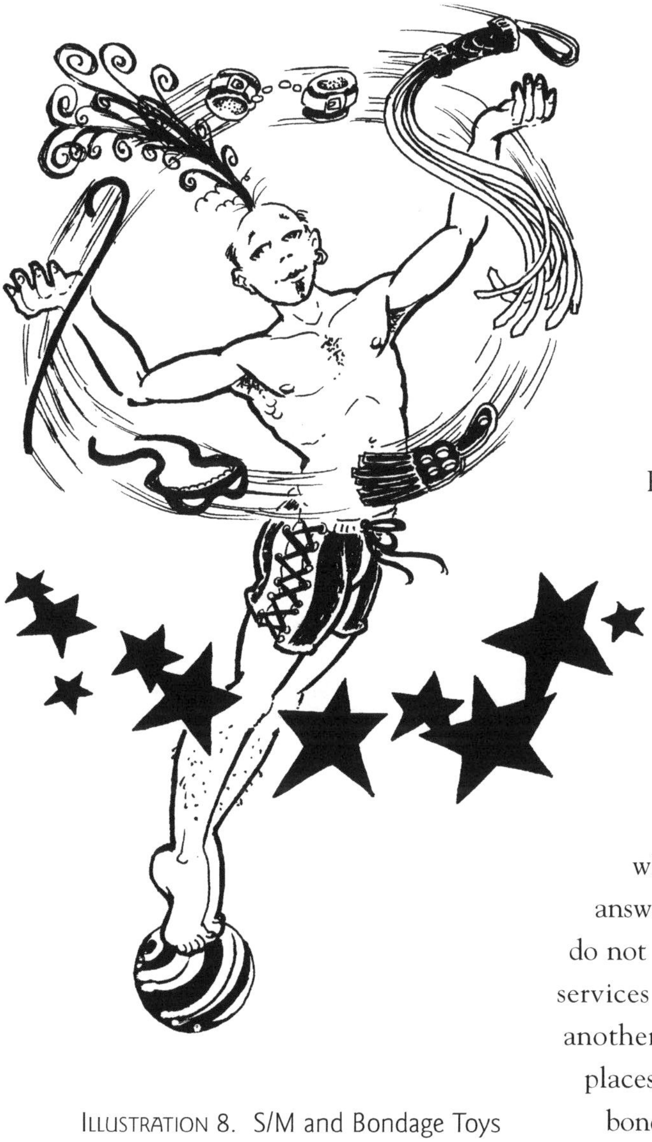

Most quality S/M retailers and mail-order operations employ educated staff who will be happy to answer your questions. If you do not feel comfortable with the services of one company, find another. There are numerous places to purchase S/M and bondage toys (see Resources).

ILLUSTRATION 8. S/M and Bondage Toys

Toys, Safer Sex, and Cleaning

To prevent infections and STDs, use condoms or other barriers on your sex toys—especially if you are going to share them. If you do not want to use barriers, do not share your toys. Wash them carefully after each use.

Condoms can be used on dildos, butt plugs, and vibrators. You can even stretch them over the large head of an electric vibrator. If you use latex on your anal toys, be sure to stretch the condom over the base of the toy so that it does not slip off up the anal canal. And if you are using plastic (not silicone) dildos and anal toys, use a condom every time you use the toy, even if you are masturbating. Plastic material is porous and absorbs dirt.

Clean your toys between uses with an antibacterial soap or a 30 percent hydrogen peroxide/water mix. You can wipe down the surface of your vibrators or other battery-operated or electric toys with alcohol or hydrogen peroxide. Test a small area first to see if the plastic material will react to the alcohol. Silicone toys can be disinfected by boiling for up to five minutes.

You can wash your leather harness and restraints with soap and water and hang them to dry. Whips and other leather goods can be wiped down with a hydrogen peroxide and water mixture and hung to dry.

Keep your sex toys in a clean, dry place. You may want to keep your dildos and plugs in separate baggies. Plastic and silicone can attract fuzzies and dust. Also, be sure your storage place is animal-proof. Dogs and cats seem to love gnawing on your favorite toys!

Erotic Books and DVDs

We now have shelves and shelves of erotic books by women. You'll find anthologies like *Best Women's Erotica* and *Best American Erotica* reviewed in the mainstream press and sold widely in bookstores. You'll still find the best selection of women's erotica at specialty stores—the same stores that sell quality sex toys designed for women. Erotic books and DVDs can offer ideas of what is possible sexually, give you fodder for fantasy, show you what you don't like, and turn you on. You can find soft erotica with subtle suggestions of sex or explicit get-down-to-it representations of sex, S/M, exhibitionism, and voyeurism. You'll find erotica intended for culturally diverse audiences—such as *Best Black Women's Erotica*, *The Oy of Sex*, a collection of Jewish women's erotica, *Juicy Mangos*, a collection of Latina erotica, and *Best Lesbian Erotica*, the annual series of lesbian and bisexual women's erotica.

You may like erotic books and DVDs that show a different sexual orientation than your preference. As a lesbian, you may like heterosexual or gay male erotica; as a heterosexual, you may like lesbian erotica. Fantasies and turn-ons often differ from how you choose to express yourself sexually.

As you begin to explore your sexuality more deeply, desires may emerge that contradict your values or political beliefs. You may get turned on by the idea of being taken or taking someone else sexually. These contradictions exist in all of us. Talk to people about them. Explore them. Don't discard them into the "bad" category—be curious about them. What do you have to discover about yourself and your sexuality by looking at these desires?

Erotica: A Journey into Women's Sexuality is an independently produced documentary that looks at the contributions of women whose artistic creations center around sex. I find many things about the film powerful. Each of the women talks about her own sexual transformation and how she evolved her self-defined sexuality and sexual expression. Candida Royalle, who writes and produces pornography, said that her work in this industry called her to look deeply at her own sexuality, the damage done to women's sexuality by our culture, and the possibility of personal healing. Annie Sprinkle shares a very poignant story about attacks on her sexually explicit performance art. One Australian radio announcer, playing tapes of speeches by Hitler, said he knew what to do with women like Annie Sprinkle, who is Jewish. This level of attack is profound. What did he find so threatening in Annie Sprinkle's representations of women's sexuality? Other women in the film speak of carving out a place for their own sexual empowerment in a society that offers little room for women's sexuality.

Many people critique pornography for its male view of sex and sexuality, and for not portraying women as viable and self-defined sexual beings. Studies also show that a high percentage of survivors of childhood sexual abuse and adult sexual assault work in the pornography and sex industry. This then begs the question of consent. If a survivor is not healing, she may still believe that the only thing about her of worth is her sexuality. Her tolerance of being used or abused sexually may be high, and there may be real poverty and oppression keeping her in the sex industry. These factors do not make for empowered consent.

> *I started dancing because sex was what I knew. I knew how to be sexual with men, how to have some control that way. I started stripping as soon as I turned eighteen. That grew into prostitution, mostly with men about my dad's age. It all seemed very familiar, too familiar.—Jody*

Many women work in the sex industry by choice, however, and do feel empowered to consent. They see women's sexual empowerment as a key to changing and healing society at large. Women in this position for the most part have the economic options to choose whether to be in the sex industry. Economic choice is a fundamental part of empowered consent.

> *I chose to do sex work for a while. I know it doesn't work for some women, but it was great for me. I felt like I controlled the situation. I got to choose what I do with my sex. Plus, I like sex and think it can be healing and powerful.—C.B.*

You may or may not like pornography. You may find yourself compelled and turned off at the same time. Lots of women shy away from porn because they don't know what they will like. To get an idea of what's available, see *The Smart Girl's Guide to Porn* and *The Ultimate Guide to Adult Videos*, both by Violet Blue. *The Ultimate Guide* features a wide selection of videos and DVDs, with ratings for woman-oriented content, lesbian content, safer sex, inclusion of people of color, chemistry between partners, and quality filmmaking.

Phone Sex

The telephone can become a sex toy in its own right. You can have sex over the telephone that can be as powerful and erotic as sex you have in person. Because some people find it easier to talk explicitly about sex over the phone than in person, phone sex can be a great way to practice your erotic talk.

> *My partner and I grew our sex life into this amazing and exciting experience using phone sex while we lived apart. It was so yummy.*—Aurora

Professional phone sex lines are also available. Most folks are familiar with these 900 numbers. Some sex talk lines are designed for callers to speak with a professional. Others are set up for callers to talk to one another, usually through a series of voice mail systems. If you choose, you can also arrange to talk live to others on the service. You can find these services advertised in the back of erotic magazines or your local weekly rag. This type of phone sex line is often free for women, while the male callers pay.

Cyber Sex

Computers may be the latest in high-tech sex toys. Numerous sites offering different types of sexual experiences can be found easily. There are sites with erotic pictures, sexually explicit chat rooms, and some offering reliable sex education. You can also shop for your sex toys online. Many of these sites, especially the ones advertising explicit photos, charge a fee for entry. Others are free. They will all post age requirement notices on their front pages.

Your Play Toys

The guiding principle here is exploration. Try out the toys, books, and DVDs that grab your attention and go with what titillates you. It is perfectly normal to feel embarrassed the first time you walk into a store that sells sex toys—or even the tenth time! It can be nerve-racking even ordering over the phone or online. The more you talk with others about sex, the more normal it will seem to make choices that support your sexual development. You'll become more comfortable with sex by engaging in the exploration of it.

Sex Guide Exercises

1. What sex toys might you like to try? How can you use sex toys to support your sexual growth?

2. Check out one of the toy stores listed in the Resources. Visit a Web site, call a mail-order company to request a catalog, or walk into a store near you.

chapter fifteen

Spiritual Sexuality

Tantra

Tantra is a sexual practice that is rooted in ancient Eastern spiritual disciplines, one of a number of such practices found in ancient Japanese, Tibetan, Chinese, Hindu, and Native American spiritual traditions. Tantra essentially combines sexuality with spirituality and treats sex as both an energetic and a potentially transcendent experience. Both the body and sexuality are considered vehicles with which to contact the sacred. Tantra has become more popular and accessible in the West in the last twenty-five years and particularly popular in the last decade. *The Art of Sexual Ecstasy* by Margot Anand does an excellent job of translating tantric practices for the Western mind. See the Bibliography for other titles as well. In a culture where sex and religion are so often considered antithetical, tantra can be a refreshing look at sex and sexuality, bringing the sacred back into sex.

Tantra teaches one to look at sex as an energetic and spiritual experience. The goal is not necessarily orgasm, but rather the opening of the body and spirit to God/Great Spirit/Vishnu/Universe. This energy can also be focused toward healing and opening the body and the sexual body. Tantric practitioners learn breath and movement patterns that increase the sexual energy in the body and the connection between partners. The focus of sex and sexual sensations is raised from the genitals to spread up the *chakra* system and over the whole body.

After a childhood of being used as a sexual object for my father, I was relieved to find tantra. It brought something pure and beautiful back to sex. It was no longer a way for someone to use me but a way for me to connect with myself, with another, and with the sacred. This has been very healing for me.—Cheryl

Yoni Massage

Yoni and lingam are the standard tantric names for the vulva and the male genitalia, respectively. Different tantric practitioners teach different ways of touching the body and genitals to raise the sexual energy. Annie Sprinkle and Joseph Kramer developed what they call the Miraculous Mooshy Massage for the Body Electric School (see Resources for contact information). This is a multistep massage process whose goal is to raise sexual energy and teach people how to touch women's bodies and genitals. The process includes full-body touch, vulva accupressure points, relaxation and breathing techniques, and spreading the erotic energy over the entire body. Most of us are thrown into the mix with little real sex education, much less instruction on how best to touch and be touched, so this is a wonderful tool to learn by.

I learned the yoni massage at a training. While this might sound out there, it was such a great experience. I got to really learn about the different parts of my own anatomy and different ways to touch and be touched sexually. I can pass this information on to my lovers now.—Jo

Sacred Masturbation and Ceremony

You do not have to practice tantra specifically to make your sexual expression sacred. Many sacred sex practices are available. Betty Dodson, in her book *Selfloving*, teaches how to create a sacred ritual for masturbation. She suggests you set up a sacred space, and moreover time, to truly care for and nourish yourself sexually.

You can create sacred space, ritual, or ceremony around sex or masturbation on your own. You might want to set up a healing ceremony or a sexual self-forgiveness ritual. You can make your masturbation a beautiful celebration and your partner sex a sacred gift.

The best definition of ceremony or ritual I have found comes from Serge Kahali King, a Hawaiian shaman, who speaks of sacred ceremony as creating an environment and intention to move or transform us. Ask yourself what moves you or is sacred or special to you. Then consider your intention. What do you want to create, heal, or bless in your ritual? Use these components to set up a sacred space or ceremony for yourself or to share with your sexual partner. Here are some ideas for creating a sacred ceremony or ritual for yourself:

Create a beautiful space. You may want to drape cloths, display special objects, light candles, burn sage or incense, put on music. Set your intention. What do you want this ceremony to celebrate? What do you want to heal in this ritual? Call in any teachers, or God/Goddess/Great Spirit, to be with you. Breathe and center, becoming present and aware of the sacred space you are creating. Take pleasure in your sacred sexuality. Poems and songs can be inspirational in starting or ending. It is lovely to share food after a ceremony.

> My partner taught me that all acts of pleasure are acts of the Spirit. What divine force would give us such a capacity for pleasure, and then say, "Don't use it"?—Akaya

Learning More

The traditions of tantra and sacred sexual practices were historically passed down through the teacher-student or guru-devotee relationship, one that is usually unfamiliar to those in the West. As tantric practices become more prevalent in the West, there are more forms of learning available. Many books, DVDs, and tapes are available on the subject, and both workshops and private consultations with practitioners and teachers can be found in many areas. Be aware that participating in workshops will include exercises in working with your sexual energy, and may include nudity. Ask the organization or trainer to give you a detailed description of the course.

As with any sexual practice, there are tantric practitioners who have more and less integrity and more and less competency with the issues of childhood sexual abuse. If wish to learn about tantra, use your own criteria to assess who you want to explore with and learn from. Just because someone talks about spirituality does not mean he or she will have the competence to support your sexual healing from childhood sexual abuse, or the appropriate boundaries to do so. Check out the credentials of workshop leaders and teachers, ask about their experience with survivors, and ask what they understand about sexual healing after childhood sexual abuse.

For more resources on tantra and sacred sexuality, please see the Resources section.

Sex Guide Exercises

1. What do you feel is sacred about sex, your body, and your sexuality?
2. What might you be interested in learning about tantra or sacred sexuality?

chapter sixteen

Intimacy and Self-Forgiveness

Mixing emotional intimacy and sex is powerful and challenging for survivors of childhood sexual abuse. You can be sure that if you are intimate both emotionally *and* sexually with your partners, the sparks of your sexual healing will light fires! This can be both exciting and tumultuous. Your history of sexual abuse will come bubbling up to the surface. Because more of you is present in your relationships, more feelings and more triggers will emerge during sex. This is not a failure, or as one survivor puts it, "the beginning of the end to yet another relationship." Rather, it is a portal into healing your sexuality.

Combining Intimacy and Sex: Turning up the Heat

Being emotionally intimate with sex partners may seem like a given by social standards. We are taught that we should to be in love before we have sex, and that sex should lead to partnership. While sex is physically intimate, it does not necessarily involve emotional or spiritual intimacy. People have sex with people they love, like, and don't know—and even with people they don't like. Sharing emotional and spiritual intimacy are only two of many reasons people have sex. Being in a relationship is no guarantee of intimacy, either. It is possible to be married or partnered for years and have very nonintimate sex.

I like having sex with friends and other people I know I am not going to get involved with. It gives me room to explore and be playful, and I get triggered a lot less.—Rebecca

I don't think I've had truly intimate sex, the gazing into each other's eyes sex, with my husband for years. Our sex has become very functional.—Jackie

Intimacy requires feeling safe and being willing to be vulnerable and more transparent than usual. You can experience an instantaneous connection with someone you've just met. Lasting intimacy, however, is built over time and involves both conflict and ease as you come to know and be known in all of your most vulnerable and imperfect aspects. Intimacy is an ongoing process of risking and revealing as you share yourself with another. The experience of intimacy can be creative and generative.

I used to think I was great at being intimate and close; then I started healing. A lot of that closeness was my survival cover, a way to feel safe and to try to be loved and loving. A lot of me wasn't there, though. I acted in a way I thought the person wanted me to, trying to fulfill their needs. Maybe they felt close, but I didn't.—Rosa

Being intimate, really vulnerable with another person is the most terrifying part of my healing. Letting myself actually depend on someone again is a big, big risk.—Louisa

In my work with survivors, I find that intimacy intensifies the risk and the vulnerability of a sexual relationship. When we are intimate with a partner, we face a greater risk of losing her or of needing him, and even of being loved. As we feel safer, the unfinished business of our abuse will enter the relationship more readily. We tend to unravel more easily in an intimate relationship.

I can get deeply sexual, into my body—let's go to it, babe—with someone until the emotional intensity of our relationship becomes greater than the sexual intensity. Then, my sexuality fades, turns off. I am looking for a time when those two will be seamless.—Akaya

The closer I get to my boyfriend, the more I want to have sex with other guys. I want sex to be easy and light. I want to be in control of it and not feel so vulnerable. Now that we are closer and I have risked more, our sex isn't like that anymore.—Shandell

For women who have been sexually abused by family members, having sex with someone who feels like "family" can seem incestuous. Making commitments, such as moving in together, can be triggering.

About four years into my relationship, my partner hit "family status" in my heart. On the one hand it was great; I was letting myself trust more deeply than I ever had. On the other hand, I did not want to have sex with my "family." I finally wanted to live in a safe house, with a safe family that I didn't have to have sex with.—Janet

It's easier to keep the sexual abuse and triggers compartmentalized when you are emotionally distant from your partner. You may find it easier to be sexual outside of intimate relationships. You may find yourself having nonintimate or "checked out" sex with someone you are emotionally very close to.

Once I get close to someone, I start to go away when we are sexual. I feel far away from them, and wonder what I ever liked about them anyway. I want to get away to feel safe.—Laura

Sex is easiest with people I hardly know.—Lourdes

Just as masturbation is a good way to get to know your sexuality, intimacy with yourself is good practice for being intimate with others. Intimacy with yourself is not about isolation. Intimacy with yourself means accompanying yourself through all of your feelings, sensations, thoughts, wackiness, and imperfections. It is getting closer to yourself. The more you can be present with yourself, the easier it will be to be present with another.

Sensitive versus Intimate

Survivors can be amazingly sensitive and receptive to other people. We've been well trained there! When you were being abused, survival hinged on your ability to pay exquisite attention to your surroundings. Being sensitive does not necessarily make you good at intimacy, however. Intimacy means being able to be fully present with yourself and another at the same time. It does not mean abandoning yourself to gain another's approval or giving up what you care about as you support your partner in his or her interests. Intimacy means being willing to experience conflict, and to use conflict to deepen your intimacy. It means risking trust with another at deeper and deeper levels over time. That part never really gets

> **How to Build Intimacy**
>
> Practice being with yourself and with another at the same time.
>
> Treat conflict as something that can build intimacy.
>
> Communicate openly and truthfully.
>
> Develop both clear boundaries and emotional flexibility.
>
> Practice self-dignity and grant your partner self-dignity, too.
>
> Affirm and acknowledge yourself and your partner regularly.
>
> Build trust.
>
> Allow support, pleasure, and conflict— all in the same relationship!
>
> Practice embodiment, emotional sourcing, and boundary exercises.
>
> Find a friend or coach to help you learn about intimacy.

comfortable. The payoff is grand, but there is no guarantee of comfort. Intimacy after childhood sexual abuse means a commitment to grow and learn; in fact, it requires the same practices and tools as those you are learning in sexual healing: embodiment, consent, openness to emotions, healing through triggers, trust, and self-forgiveness. I encourage survivors to find a coach, therapist, or friend who is good at relationships and to learn from that person. Keep educating yourself.

Self-Forgiveness

Forgiving myself and being forgiven by a community of people who love me was the most moving thing that I have experienced in my healing process. I feel like

I have permission to live now. It is all right that I made it out alive; in fact, it is wonderful that I did!—Carla

Many folks think forgiving the perpetrator is the final step in healing from childhood sexual abuse. You may have been told this is the goal of your healing process. Forgiving the perpetrator may naturally arise as a by-product of your own healing, but in my experience it is not necessarily the goal. If you do feel forgiveness, warmth, and compassion for your perpetrator, welcome that as a piece of your own heart thawing. But keep in mind that your healing lies in feeling at least that much love, warmth, and compassion *for yourself.*

When I remembered, the first thing I said was, "My dad is lucky he has such a forgiving daughter. I forgive him. I am done with that." That was my way of repressing the pain. I then spent the next two years in excruciating pain, wondering what was wrong with me, why I was so fucked up and miserable.—Janet

Forgiving yourself is paramount. Survivors internalize the blame for sexual abuse. This makes sense when viewed in the context of children's developmental process. Children have not fully differentiated themselves from other people and so attempt to make sense of the world by relating outside events to their own behavior. To small children, the whole world is about them. Kids think they caused their parents' divorce because they spilled their milk or wouldn't go to bed on time. This is the same thinking that goes into believing that sexual abuse was in some way your fault.

I spent most of my childhood trying to figure out what I could do differently to make the abuse stop. I was very, very good, trying to control all my behaviors, trying to do whatever my parents wanted. I figured if I could be perfect then he'd have no reason to hurt me anymore. The rules kept changing, though.—Naomi

The social system perpetuates the view that sexual abuse is the fault of the child. Too often, adults demand of children, "What did you do to make him do that?" or "Are you sure that happened?" Much like adult rape victims who face a criminal justice system that questions the length of their skirts instead of protecting women from sexual violence, children who report sexual abuse are often met with blame and disbelief.

Many women who were abused as children also feel survivor's guilt. *Why was I the one to survive? Why did I make it out when my younger brother didn't? Why am I healing when my big sister is institutionalized? Why do I deserve to be okay?* This can be particularly intense for survivors of multiple victim abuse and ritual abuse. Any abuse setting in which other victims either literally or figuratively didn't make it can produce tremendous guilt for the surviving party.

> *I survived the ritual abuse and others didn't. I have carried tremendous guilt for that. I wondered, Why me? Why am I the one who made it out?*—Carol

Self-forgiveness is directly tied to how much pleasure, sexual expression, and intimacy you will allow yourself in your life. If you are punishing yourself for being "bad" or "dirty," why would you allow yourself to delight in sexual expression? Self-forgiveness is the doorway through which you move toward what you want in your life.

Sexual abuse may have been your only source of affection or touch. We all need physical contact with other humans as much as we need water, food, and air. In the case of children who receive no other physical affection, any touch is a relief.

> *I sometimes hate myself for having sought out his touch. I was starving. I figured if this is the way I can get love and affection, I'll take it.*—Jo

Let Yourself off the Hook

You can take steps to forgive yourself. First, explore why you think you are at fault. Become familiar with these beliefs. You don't have to contradict them or prove to yourself that they aren't true. Just look at what you truly believe about the abuse. One survivor wrote, "I think that the abuse is my fault because I was sexy even at six years old." Do you blame yourself because you didn't fight back? Because you minimized the abuse? Include it all. You are probably not alone in your reasons for thinking the abuse was your fault.

Many survivors use their sexual desires as justification for their self-blame. One survivor wrote: "I think that the abuse is my fault because I like anal sex today; that is one of the ways I was abused, so I must have liked it then." Another wrote, "I am into kinky sex. Maybe I am just as perverted as my perps." Explore this for yourself.

As you face what you believe is your fault, check in with people you trust. Do your close friends think the abuse was your fault because you liked getting attention? Or because you're doing better than your little sister? This reality check is essential in developing a reasonable set of expectations for the girl that you were.

People will want to use arguments to convince you that the abuse was not your fault. The experience of self-blame is profoundly deep, however. You can understand intellectually you are not at fault, but that may not change how deeply you blame yourself.

The next step is to begin an active process of forgiving yourself. To do this, you don't have to believe the abuse was not your fault. Self-forgiveness is granted, not earned. You can believe you are to blame *and* forgive yourself. "It's my fault because I wasn't smart enough to figure out how to make it stop, and I am forgivable." "I asked my dad to touch me, and I can forgive myself for that." Look at your reasons for thinking the abuse was your fault. Point by point, practice forgiving yourself. Say aloud to yourself, "X may be true *and* I forgive myself.

The sexual abuse was my fault because...

Here's what some survivors in a workshop came up with:

- I was too smart.

- I wasn't smart enough.

- I had an orgasm.

- I like kinky sex.

- I asked for our "special time."

- I abused my little brother, so I am just as bad.

- He didn't really mean it; I am blowing it out of proportion.

- Women don't really sexually abuse kids.

- He was abused, too, so it doesn't count.

- I'm gay.

- I liked the attention.

- I didn't say "no."

I am so sorry this happened to me."
Write these phrases down and post
them on your bathroom mirror.
Grant yourself self-forgiveness.

The final step is to ask a trusted
friend to witness you in this
process. Ask your friend or therapist to listen as you list all of the
aspects of your history that you feel
are unforgivable. What is it like to

> ### I Am Different from My Perps Because...
>
> You are not your perpetrators, no matter what
> you enjoy sexually. Make a list of all the ways
> you are different from those who abused you.
> This list can assist you in seeing yourself and
> your choices more clearly. Start with "I choose
> to heal." Most likely, if your abuser had made
> that choice, you would not have been abused.

feel another person witnessing you? Does this person hold you responsible? Does
this person forgive you? Are you forgivable? I can assure you that everything that
you have done to survive is forgivable, no matter how terrible it seems to you.

> My brother would give me choices as to the ways that he would molest me. I
> had to pick whether he would touch my vagina and put things in it or put his
> penis in my mouth. He would end up doing whatever he wanted, but I felt like
> I picked my own demise.—Donna

> The hardest thing I have had to face was the unforgivable act of molesting a
> child that I baby-sat. I couldn't stop what I was doing. I felt so out of control.
> I thought I was going to die facing this. How could I have done this when I
> knew how horrible it was for me? I am beginning to have compassion for
> myself. I'm wondering if I will try to find the girl to apologize. I don't know if
> this will be helpful or not. What has helped me the most is talking to a few very
> close people about what I did. They felt the pain with me, and helped me feel
> compassion for myself and the trap I lived in.—Danielle

Self-Trust and Compassion

How can you learn to trust yourself, your decisions, and your sexual energy? You
can rebuild trust with yourself by acting on your own behalf over time. If you need

to forgive yourself for not taking care of yourself, do so by learning how to take care of yourself now. If you do not trust yourself to have sexual boundaries, say so. Acknowledge that this is a problem and learn how to develop sexual boundaries that serve you. Self-trust involves the intention to do right by yourself, consistent action to back that up, and the capacity to know how to take that action.

A childhood of sexual abuse does not prepare you well for life. You may find yourself lacking basic skills to take good care of yourself. That you survived to adulthood is both a blessing and a challenge. You may feel like a little girl, but as an adult you are now responsible for your own well-being. Survivors are very creative people when it comes to staying alive in spite of trauma. Now is the time to channel this creativity into learning to live well.

This is where compassion for yourself comes in. Even if all your survival skills now prove self-destructive—skills like denying your desires, checking out during sex, or avoiding intimacy—give yourself credit for developing these skills when you needed them. And give yourself a break for not knowing what you don't know. What are the problem areas in your life? What things can't you manage? You may not know how to make friends, maintain sexual relationships, find employment that nurtures your creativity, or have an orgasm. What skills do you need to learn? Whom can you learn from? How about a book, a friend, a workshop, or a teacher? You are not deficient for not knowing how to do even the "simplest" things. If you do not know how, it is because you were not taught. You can learn how to take care of yourself and to build the life you want.

It is about learning how to surrender again, this time to my own goodness and trustworthiness—Aurora

Do I Deserve Pleasure?

The more I forgive myself, the more pleasure I allow myself... Now I give myself permission to have in my life those things that bring me pleasure. I am spending less time "making up" for being abused by suffering.—Cheryl

Many survivors feel that they should pay for what happened to them as children. You may believe that you need to suffer to make up for being bad, dirty, or wrong. You may think that because others are suffering you should as well, that you would betray those who are in pain by having pleasure. Chances are that nothing in your life prepared you for pleasure or the belief that you deserve it. When you feel pleasure, you may feel guilty or ashamed.

You deserve and always did deserve pleasure. You deserve and always did deserve a life in which your well-being is respected. You are deserving just because you are alive. Do you wish more pleasure for others? Include yourself in this well-wishing.

Pleasure

Many survivors are unfamiliar with both emotional and sexual pleasure. Pleasure can be scary and strange, and therefore suspect. Many survivors have spent their entire lives dealing with profound pain. Pain, lack, and betrayal are familiar and therefore "safe." When in your history was it safe to feel pleasure? When could you relax enough to feel at ease in your body?

Reclaiming pleasure is like letting water back into a sea sponge that has been dried for years and is hard and crusty. The sponge initially repels the water and then very slowly begins to let it in. First, a little water seeps in around the edges, and then slowly the water reaches deeper into the sponge. Eventually, with a steady supply of water, the sponge becomes supple and pliable again, able to easily let water in and squeeze it out.

Of course, if you leave the sponge out to dry, it will harden again. To keep it supple, you must regularly submerge that sponge in water. Similarly, if you are denied pleasure, you will learn to resist pleasure. To learn how to embody pleasure in your life, you'll have to practice taking in pleasure, little by little, over and over again. This may be terrifying. Don't worry; you can go at your own pace.

What brings you pleasure? What give you physical joy? Emotional joy? What can you do to incorporate more of what is pleasurable to you into your life? What can you do that will allow pleasure into your body? Into your emotional repertoire?

Self-Permission

You may need to officially and overtly give yourself permission to experience pleasure, intimacy, sexual expression, and satisfaction. What would your sex life be like if you gave yourself permission to have it all? To not settle for anything less than everything you want?

I give myself permission, because really it's not up to anyone else. My body, my life, and my sex are mine and no one else's. This is the only life I have; I'm going to live it fully to my own standards.—Anna

From this moment forward you have permission to fully express your sexuality. You are granted permission to experience pleasure, delight, intensity—whatever you want. You have full permission to have your boundaries, needs, and desires. How's that? Granting yourself permission to be fully expressed sexually is a courageous act. Go for it.

Personal and community support are as important as ever in this stage of the process. Find at least one other person who is as excited as you about you having a fully expressed sexuality. When things get tough, ask your friend to remind you just why you want a sex life, anyway.

What keeps you from granting yourself permission to have the sexuality and sexual expression you want, on your own terms? Do you feel you need someone else's permission? Who might that be? Your parents? God?

Whom do I need permission from to be fully expressed sexually? I'm not sure. Maybe God? Somehow I am "bad" or "damaged" still, so I am not allowed to fully be my big, bright self.—Roslyn

Some survivors do not feel safe enough to give themselves permission to express themselves sexually. When you were being abused, it was not safe to reveal yourself or to express your sexuality in your own way.

Explore all the nooks and crannies of your life in which you don't give yourself permission to fully be yourself. How does it serve you to deny aspects of yourself? Are you keeping yourself hidden, punished, or safe? What would it feel like to be both safe and fully expressed sexually?

For me it is about safety. It has never been safe to come out all the way. I sneak around, letting a little of me come out here, letting a different part of me out there...Now the people in my life would probably rather I be my whole self.
—Cindy

You now have the power to choose sexual partners and friends who respect you, support your growth, and delight in your successes. They may even want to join you in your adventure by doing some sexual healing of their own!

Sexual Expression Permission Slip

Write yourself a permission slip to have the sex life you want. Here is a sample. Of course, you can create your own permission slip, using language that is meaningful for you. If you need permission from others, or from God, write yourself a permission slip from them. List all the specific expressions, acts, and feelings you want to receive explicit permission for.

I, _____ , give myself complete permission to be fully expressed sexually on my own terms. This includes expressing myself sexually in whatever ways, wherever, whenever, and with whomever I choose from this day forward.

Specifically, I give myself full permission

- to have the boundaries that I want and need sexually.

- to acknowledge all of my feelings while I am being sexual, and to take care of them in whatever way best serves me in the given situation.

- to laugh during sex.

- to masturbate.

- to be sexually brazen or shy.

- to be in my body.

- to say "yes," "maybe," or "no" to sex.

- to do that one thing I've never told anyone that I've always wanted to do sexually, like...

You, _____, are granted full permission to express yourself sexually on your own terms. You have my blessings.

Enjoy!

Lovingly,

(your signature)

Sex Guide Exercises

1. Make a list of all of the things related to the abuse that you believe are your fault. Then read the list to yourself. Look at it. Do this every day for a week, a month, or a year. What would you say to a little girl who told you these things about herself? What would you feel for her?

2. Read that same list to your therapist, a friend, or your partner. Let that person witness you and confirm that you are forgiven. Ask that person to tell you whatever you need to hear to feel supported in forgiving yourself.

3. Write about what your sex life would be like if you were completely forgiven.

4. The following exercise can help you increase your tolerance for intimacy with a partner:

    a. Sit in a comfortable position, facing your partner. Sit upright so that you are alert. Breathe down into your belly, letting the air fill your belly and chest. Look into your partner's face and eyes. Continue to breathe. Notice what happens in your body. Sit in your own experience while being connected with your partner. Try not to be in your partner's experience, attempting to figure out what he or she is feeling. Be in your body.

    b. After three minutes, each of you can tell the other what you notice in your body. What sensations are there? Were you able to stay present? Where did you float off to? And when?

    c. Then gaze at each other for another three minutes. What is different now? What do you notice?

    d. Talk about the experience.

    e. If you want to up the ante, try doing this exercise while nude.

chapter seventeen

Partnering with Survivors of Sexual Abuse

It's Not Your Fault

One of the most difficult things for partners is remembering that your lover's pain is not your fault. When you are in it for the long haul with someone healing from childhood sexual abuse, her pain will come out around you and at you. You can count on it. When your lover gets upset during sex, you may feel tempted to take responsibility. You may think you triggered her, and that she wouldn't be in pain if you hadn't said X or if you hadn't done Y. Not true. Even if something you said or did triggered her, the feelings that emerged were there, waiting to come out. They were *her* feelings.

Understandably, you don't want your lover to be in emotional pain. The pain of recovery is essential to healing, though. You can't heal from childhood sexual abuse without feeling the emotions associated with the trauma.

As a partner of a survivor, be aware of the inclination to suppress your own emotions and communications to avoid triggering her. Although editing your thoughts, feelings, desires, and speech may help her sidestep short-term pain, it is a setup for both of you. What you do or say may, in fact, trigger her, but she can handle it. Even in her moments of greatest emotional turmoil, don't overlook her courage and empowerment. Treat her with care *and* with dignity. Avoiding triggers is not any healthier for you than it is for her!

You can support your lover, but you can't fix her or make the effects of the abuse go away. Over and over again, I have heard survivors say that what they want most is a witness, someone who is willing and able to sit with them in their story. If you can offer this, you are giving your partner a priceless gift.

No Saviors, No Patients

You are not a savior, and your lover is not a patient. Your lover is not broken or hurt, and it is not your job to rescue her. When partners get stuck in savior/patient roles, they are both ultimately disempowered. The truth is, you are both incredibly courageous to be engaging in the healing of abuse. So many survivors and partners stay in denial about it instead. Acknowledge yourselves and each other for this.

It will help you to learn something about childhood sexual abuse. The patterns of abuse, experiences of survivors, and recovery process are fairly well mapped out in books like *The Courage to Heal* by Ellen Bass and Laura Davis and *Trauma and Recovery* by Judith Lewis Herman. It's much easier to avoid pitfalls such as savior/patient roles when you know what's going on.

Practice viewing each other as whole human beings. Tell each other regularly what you appreciate about the other. Talk about the wholeness, vulnerability, and innate sense of power or wisdom you see in each other. Give yourself lots of kudos for hanging in there. No patients or saviors are needed here.

Take Care of Yourself

As a partner of a survivor, you need to be very attentive to your own needs. An often-made mistake for partners of survivors is giving to the point of depletion because the situation seems to call for it. Learning to recognize, negotiate, and care for your needs will serve (and potentially save) your relationship.

Incest and childhood sexual abuse is horrible, and in many ways it is a personal and social crisis. Yet if the survivor is out of immediate danger, the emergency is over. The healing process takes time. From the initial "crisis stage," when she begins to face the effects of the abuse, you can count on at least two years of focused healing before things stabilize. Recovery from childhood sexual abuse takes a long time (some would say it is a lifelong process), but over time her abuse issues will take up less and less space in her life. If you are involved with a survivor, childhood sexual abuse and its implications will be a part of your relationship. This path can be both arduous and deeply beautiful.

Consider getting support for yourself as well. You can turn to friends or a counselor—just make sure they are educated about the process of healing from childhood sexual abuse. Books like *Allies in Healing* by Laura Davis can also help.

Continue to do the things that you enjoy. Whether you pursue a hobby, create art, play sports, or hang out with your friends, make time for the things that give your life meaning. This will be a place of balance and renewal for you, and help bring joy to your relationship.

Expand Your Sexual Repertoire

Aspects of your lover's healing naturally will emerge in sex. While this can be trying, it can also be a powerful way to build intimacy. By sharing your deep, shadow places you can build incredible trust. Sexual healing can be a great opportunity for you to grow and develop sexually, too.

We live in a sex-negative culture. We all could benefit from some sexual healing. At the very least, we all could learn more about sex. In what ways would you like to grow sexually? How would you like to develop your capacity for intimacy?

Although you may be tempted, don't build a sex life around triggers. Both you and your survivor partner will need to learn to tolerate a full range of emotions, including the pain that is a part of this recovery. Think of the fear and pain as healing, not as something to be avoided. Keep coming back to expressing your full sexuality. This may not be possible at the moment, but it is the ultimate intention of recovery. Read chapter 11 on triggers with your partner, and design a trigger plan for your sex life.

You and your partner may have different sexual needs and desires. Contrary to what you might expect, it is not always the case that the survivor doesn't want to have sex. You may want a break from sex. If one of you does not want to be sexual, negotiate this clearly. Do you want to take a three-week break? A three-month break? What types of healing work can you commit to in the meantime? When will you reassess your agreement?

As your lover heals, she will change. Her sexuality will evolve. You may feel as if you have a new sexual partner on your hands. Give yourself time to adjust. Be creative. How can you invent sexual experiences that work for both of you? How can you both use this as a time to grow sexually? How can you learn together?

Use the "Yes," "No," "Maybe" exercise in chapter 2 to come up with a repertoire of sensual and sexual expressions that are interesting to both of you. Explore your lists of likes, dislikes, and possible new explorations. Expand your range of what you consider pleasurable and erotic. Get away from the idea that the way you used to have sex is the only way that counts.

You Get to Change, Too

When your partner is healing sexually, you change, too. In a way, you inherit her history and her recovery process. You'll get a close-up look at what human beings can do to each other. This may call into question your basic beliefs about people and societies. How could this happen? Why is this *still* happening? What can I do? Partners go through their own stages of denial, shock, feeling, and integrating the trauma. It is normal to get angry at those who harmed your partner and to grieve the losses she has suffered as a result of the abuse.

Sharing this time with your lover can have an uncanny way of exposing your own ghosts. You may find yourself rehashing old wounds or coming up against issues you thought you had successfully avoided. Your lover and you can learn much together. What would it be like for *both* of you to be fully embodied, emotionally flexible, and sexually expressed?

Survivors as Partners

You may both be survivors of childhood sexual abuse. As you might suspect, there are unique benefits and challenges to this.

The challenges come in having appropriate boundaries and building self-referential lives. While it's great to be understood, the lines between whose stuff is whose can get blurry. The best bet is to focus on and take full responsibility for your own healing. Let your partner take full responsibility for his or hers. Do not push your partner to take your path to healing. Your road is yours only.

The benefit is, of course, a great understanding. There is so much you do not have to explain. You'll both be familiar with the intricacies of abuse and healing. You can support each other in committing to each other's recovery, and you can share the process in many ways.

Sex Guide Exercises

1. If you are inclined to feel responsible for your lover's triggers and emotions, take a moment now to differentiate between your behaviors and intentions and those of the people who harmed her. Are her feelings about you or them?

2. Sit down with your partner and talk about your commitment to sexual healing and to each other. *Why heal sexually, anyway? Why go through this together? What do we have to gain? How might this process change us for the better? What parts of ourselves or our relationship might we have to leave behind?*

3. Take a few minutes each week to practice appreciating your partner. Sit comfortably, facing your partner. Settle into your body. Practice your emotional sourcing. Find that place in you that makes you feel grounded and at peace. For three minutes, tell your partner what you love and cherish about her. What are her virtues? When the three minutes are up, you can switch, and your partner can tell you what she loves and cherishes about you. As you listen to her appreciation, relax. Letting her appreciation really sink in shows your partner respect.

4. Make a pleasure date with your partner. Take a break from emotional issues and healing, and focus on having fun. You could do something together as

simple as taking a walk, going to a movie, or working in the garden. Settle into being together and enjoying time with each other. Keep this as a regular practice throughout the sexual healing process.

chapter eighteen

Your Powerful Sexual Self: Who Are You Becoming?

Visions of where we are going are always out in front of us. As we attain one goal, a new one stretches ahead to draw us onward. As you progress in healing, your ideas about your new sexuality will change. A new dream may emerge. Or you may realize midstream that what you thought you wanted isn't really what you want anymore. Your vision will change and grow over time.

What will your empowered sexual self look, sound, and feel like?

You may take for granted that sex is a normal and healthy part of being human. You could be embodied and at choice sexually, knowing and practicing healthful boundaries. You may be able to communicate your desires and fantasies to your partners. Ideally, you will practice safer sex; you may even practice sacred sex. You could be self-referential in your sexuality, while honoring your connections with others. You may become comfortable with the contradictory nature of sex and come to accept your own sexual evolution—all of it, both the pleasure and the pain. It is up to you. What would a compelling sex life look like to you? Who do you want to become sexually?

Along the way, develop some interim goals for yourself. Maybe your dream is to become fully embodied sexually. You may have just begun to feel your body. An interim goal might be staying present while masturbating or staying present in one part of your body while you are having sex with a partner. You can set the goal of learning how you dissociate during sex and catching yourself sooner. Build lots of acknowledgment and successes into your journey.

How far in the future do you see yourself reaching your goals? How much of your sexuality resembles your vision already? What are the immediate next steps on the road to your vision? What can you do today? Tomorrow? Next week?

Let yourself be a novice. You are an apprentice, a trainee on your way to becoming the woman of your vision. Learning anything new takes practice. You'll need lots of freedom to make mistakes.

In developing a vision for your sexual healing, remember that yours will be a dynamic vision. It will change over time as you grow. You do not need rigid goals or trials that you can fail. You need a vision of your empowered sexual self that will serve as a source of encouragement, a reminder of your desires and your ability to grow and expand.

In my sexual healing workshops, I ask participants to create three visions of who they want to become sexually. If you had three full lives to live, and each could

---

Your Powerful Sexual Self

Following is a sampling of visions from workshop participants:

I am my sexuality and it is me. It isn't something split off from me any longer. There is not a lot of difference between my sexual energy and my life energy. This doesn't mean everything is sexualized, rather, everything is erotic and alive with a kind of vitality. My integrated sensual and sexual energy feeds my whole life. Sometimes I also want a break from sex. I don't want to share that energy with others. I want to pull it into myself, and sit quietly with it. It feels very peaceful.

I want to become an S/M top. I am intrigued and excited. The woman I want to become is powerful in her sexuality and awake. She dreams with other people about desire and pushing the edge, and then makes those dreams a reality. She is gentle in a very deep way. Not careful—bold. She reveals herself deeply and is willing to be vulnerable and naked in her desires. She is not afraid to go into the reaches of sex and sexuality. She is very clear with boundaries and has intimacy and a lot of play in her life. She is sexy, too.

I envision a life with a committed sexual partner, a woman. We share deeply and use sex as a way to grow. I will be scared sometimes about intimacy and how deep I can go, but I will not retreat. I'll use intimacy as a place to heal. I will learn about loss, joy, grief, birth, death, and change in sex and intimacy. I don't know how to explain it that well, but it's like taking the risk over and over again to be close with myself and close with her. Sometimes it will be easy and sometimes it will be hard, but I'll show up. This is the sexuality I want.

express a different sexual self, what would those sexualities be? Imagining three lives, rather than one, helps to get around the self-censors that tell us who we are "allowed" to become sexually—as well as the little voice that tells us our dreams are impossible. Creating three visions can also help you notice patterns in your desires. You may find that there is one form of sexual expression that comes up repeatedly. This is a strong desire, one worth paying attention to.

Be creative and outrageous. Once you have created your three visions, consider the following questions: In your visions of yourself, are you embodied? How do you embody your sexuality? How do you feel about your body? Who are your partner(s)? Is there a spiritual component to your sexuality? If so, what is it? What type of intensity do you like sexually? What kind of sex do you like? What are your powers and virtues? Does your sex life feed energy into other parts of your life?

You can write about your new sexual self in a journal or create a collage or other art piece to depict it. The more creativity you bring to this exercise, the better. Whatever medium you choose, create an external representation of your vision so that it can exist outside of your own thoughts. Display your creation where you can see it regularly. This can help keep you oriented toward your dreams.

Take a look at the woman you wish to become. How did she get to be who she is? What was her path? Keep her in your thoughts. She will have plenty to tell you.

chapter nineteen

Bibliography and Resources

TRAUMA

Childhood Sexual Abuse

BOOKS

Abused Boys: The Neglected Victims of Sexual Abuse by Mic Hunter (Ballantine Books, 1991).

Beginning to Heal: A First Book for Men and Women Who Were Sexually Abused as Children by Ellen Bass and Laura Davis (Quill, 2003).

The Betrayal Bond by Patrick J. Carnes (HCI, 1997).

Betrayal Trauma: The Logic of Forgetting Childhood Abuse by Jennifer Freyd (Harvard University Press, 1998).

Breaking Ritual Silence: An Anthology of Ritual Abuse Survivor's Stories edited by Jeanne Marie Lorena and Paula Levy (Trout and Sons, Inc., 1998).

Conspiracy of Silence: The Trauma of Incest by Sandra Butler (Volcano Press, 1996).

The Courage to Heal: A Guide for Women Survivors of Child Sexual Abuse by Ellen Bass and Laura Davis (HarperCollins, 2008).

The Courage to Heal Workbook by Laura Davis (HarperCollins, 1990).

Crossing the Boundary: Black Women Survive Incest by Melba Wilson (Seal Press, 1993).

Getting Home Alive by Aurora Levins Morales and Rosario Morales (Firebrand Books, 1986).

Healing Sex: The Complete Guide to Sexual Wholeness by Staci Haines (DVD by SIR Productions, 2004).

Healing Sex: A Mind-Body Approach to Healing Sexual Trauma by Staci Haines (Cleis Press, 2007).

Healing Your Sexual Self by Janet G. Woititz (Health Communications, Inc., 1989).

Incest, Work, and Women: Understanding the Consequences of Incest on Women's Careers, Work, and Dreams by Lesliebeth Berger (Charles C. Thomas Publisher, 1998).

No Secrets, No Lies: How Black Families Can Heal from Sexual Abuse by Robin D. Stone (Broadway, 2004).

Preventing Child Sexual Abuse: Sharing the Responsibility by Sandy K. Wurtele and Cindy L. Miller-Perrin (University of Nebraska Press, 1992).

Repressed Memories: A Journey to Recovery from Sexual Abuse by Renee Fredrickson (Simon and Schuster, 1992).

Resolving Childhood Trauma: A Long-Term Study of Abuse Survivors by Catherine Cameron (Sage Publications, 2000).

Ritual Abuse: Definitions, Glossary, the Use of Mind Control by the Los Angeles County Commission for Women (1989).

Childhood Sexual Abuse (cont.)

BOOKS (cont.)

Rocking the Cradle of Sexual Politics: What Happened When Women Said Incest by Louise Armstrong (Addison-Wesley Publishing Company, 1994).

Safe Passage to Healing: A Guide for Survivors of Ritual Abuse by Chrystine Oksana (Harper Perennial, 1994).

Sexual Abuse in Nine North American Cultures edited by Lisa Aronson Fontes (Sage Press, 1995).

The Sexual Healing Journey: A Guide for Survivors of Sexual Abuse by Wendy Maltz (HarperCollins, 2001).

Shining Through: Pulling It Together After Sexual Abuse by Bailey Leslie Wright and Mindy B. Loiselle (Safer Society Press, 1997).

Sibling Abuse: Hidden Physical, Emotional, and Sexual Trauma by Vernon Wiehe (Sage Press, 1997).

Soul Survivors: A New Beginning for Adults Abused as Children by Patrick J. Gannon (Simon and Schuster, 1992).

Strong at the Broken Places: Building Resiliency in Survivors of Trauma by Linda Sanford (Neari Press, 2005).

Thou Shalt Not Be Aware: Society's Betrayal of the Child by Alice Miller (Farrar, Straus and Giroux, 1998).

Victims No Longer: Men Recovering from Incest and Other Sexual Child Abuse by Mike Lew (Perennial, 1990).

Virginia Woolf: The Impact of Child Sexual Abuse on Her Life and Work by Louise DeSalvo (Women's Press Ltd., 1991).

When Survivors Give Birth: Understanding and Healing the Effects of Early Sexual Abuse on Childbearing Women by Penny Simkin and Phyllis Klaus (Classic Day Publishing, 2004).

Women's Sexuality After Childhood Incest by Elaine Westerlund (W.W. Norton, 1992).

Childhood Sexual Abuse (cont.)

WEB SITES

American Professional Society on the Abuse of Children (APSAC)
An interdisciplinary professional society for people working in the field of child abuse.
P.O. Box 30669
Charleston, SC 29417
(877) 40A-PSAC
apsac.fmhi.usf.edu

Childhelp
A 24-hour child abuse hotline. Trained crisis counselors provide crisis intervention, information, and referrals.
(800) 4-A-CHILD
www.childhelp.org

generation FIVE
Generation FIVE's mission is to end the sexual abuse of children within five generations. Through survivor and bystander leadership development, community prevention and intervention, public education and action, and cross-movement building, generation FIVE works to interrupt and mend the intergenerational impact of child sexual abuse on individuals, families, and communities. Rather than perpetuate the isolation of this issue, we integrate child sexual abuse prevention into social movements and community organizing targeting family violence, economic and racial oppression, and gender, age-based, and cultural discrimination. It is our belief that meaningful community response is the key to effective prevention.
3288 21st Street, #171
San Francisco, CA 94110
(415) 861-6658
Fax: (415) 861-6659
Email: info@generationFIVE.org
www.generationFIVE.org

Jim Hopper Child Sexual Abuse Resource Page
Extensive resource page with information for men and women, child sexual abuse statistics on boys and girls, and links to research, healing resources, and articles on abuse and abuse prevention.
www.jimhopper.com

The Kempe Center (The C. Henry Kempe Center for the Prevention and Treatment of Child Abuse and Neglect)
Nationally known institute. Offers model programs for treatment of children, offenders, and families. Resource library. Offers professional training.
1825 Marion Street
Denver, CO 80218
(303) 864-5300
www.kempecenter.org

MaleSurvivor
MaleSurvivor conducts research, education, advocacy, and activism to promote prevention, treatment, and elimination of sexual abuse of male children and adults. MaleSurvivor also coordinates and conducts regional retreats for male survivors and holds an annual conference that includes programming and material for survivors and their loved ones, clinicians, researchers, criminologists, attorneys, educators, clergy, law enforcement and corrections personnel, and students. MaleSurvivor also provides online chat rooms that allow survivors and professionals to talk to each other.
PMB 103, 5505 Connecticut Avenue NW
Washington, DC 20015-2601
Toll free: (800) 738-4181
www.malesurvivor.org

Childhood Sexual Abuse (cont.)

WEB SITES (cont.)

National Children's Advocacy Center

210 Pratt Avenue
Huntsville, AL 35801
(256) 533-KIDS
www.nationalcac.org

National Hopeline Network (NHN)

NHN was activated in May of 1999 to automatically connect callers—people who are depressed or suicidal, or those who are concerned about someone they love—to a certified crisis center. Trained counselors answer crisis center calls 24 hours a day, seven days a week. Callers should never encounter a busy signal or voice mail.

Hotline: (800) SUICIDE (800-784-2433)
www.hopeline.com

National Organization for Victim Assistance (NOVA)

NOVA is a private, nonprofit network of victim and witness assistance programs and practitioners, criminal justice agencies and professionals, mental health professionals, researchers, former victims, survivors, and others committed to the integration and implementation of victim rights and services. NOVA provides direct service to victims and communities that need assistance. One may call NOVA's hotline 24 hours a day for information, referrals in one's local area, or emotional support. NOVA is the oldest national group of its kind in the worldwide victim's movement.

510 King Street, Suite 424
Alexandria, VA 22314
(703) 535-6682
Hotline: (800) TRY-NOVA (800-879-6682)
www.try-nova.org

National Sexual Violence Resource Center (NSVRC)

National Sexual Violence Resource Center opened in July 2000 as a vital new center for information, resources, and research related to all aspects of sexual violence. It serves and supports state and territory coalitions, local rape crisis centers, government and tribal entities, universities, researchers, and the general public. With a large and growing library of resources, the NSVRC responds to requests for information and augments grassroots efforts to end sexual violence by distributing information and materials, including prevention tools. It coordinates efforts with other organizations and projects; provides technical assistance and customized information packets on specific topics; and maintains a Web site of current information on conferences, funding opportunities, research, and Sexual Assault Awareness Month (SAAM). The NSVRC produces a semiannual newsletter, The Resource, and booklets that focus on underserved populations. As a project of the Pennsylvania Coalition Against Rape (PCAR), the NSVRC provides resources and identifies emerging issues related to the difficult task of ending sexual violence.

123 North Enola Drive
Enola, PA 17025
Toll-free: (877) 739-3895
www.nsvrc.org

Childhood Sexual Abuse (cont.)

WEB SITES (cont.)

Raksha, Inc.: Break the Silence Project
Raksha—meaning "protection" in several
South Asian languages—is a Georgia-based
nonprofit organization for the South Asian
community. Raksha's mission is to promote a
stronger and healthier South Asian community through confidential support services,
education, and advocacy. Guided by values of
consensus in decision making, diversity in
leadership, and the dignity and worth of
every individual, Raksha strives to empower
and serve the South Asian community.
Raksha's Break the Silence Project is a com-
munity-based initiative to address Child
Sexual Abuse (CSA) in the South Asian
community. BSP is driven by a community
collective of survivors and allies under a guiding framework of community and bystander
accountability, violence prevention, social
justice, and resiliency in the face of trauma to
address the impact of CSA.
   (404) 876-0670
   Toll-free: (866) 725-7423
   Help line: (404) 842-0725
   www.Raksha.org

**Rape, Abuse & Incest National Network
(RAINN)**
RAINN, a nonprofit organization, operates
America's only national hotline for victims of
sexual assault. The hotline offers free, confidential counseling and support twenty-four
hours a day, from anywhere in the country.
The hotline is a partnership of nearly nine
hundred rape crisis centers across the country.
Callers are automatically connected to their
local center for immediate help. If a caller is
under age eighteen and chooses to share personally identifying information with the
counselor, the counselor will be mandated to
notify authorities of the sexual assault of a
minor. Only in this situation—when a minor
calls and reveals identifying information—
does the pledge of confidentiality not apply.
   2000 L Street NW, Suite 406
   Washington, DC 20036
   Hotline: (800) 656-HOPE (800-656-4673)
   Fax: (202) 544-3556
   Email: info@rainn.org
   www.rainn.org

Childhood Sexual Abuse (cont.)

WEB SITES (cont.)

Stop It Now!

Stop It Now! is a national, public health–based organization working to prevent and ultimately eradicate child sexual abuse. Through its public education, public policy, and research programs, Stop It Now! challenges abusers and people at risk for abusing to stop abusive behaviors and to reach out for help. They educate adults about how to prevent child sexual abuse and promote policy changes at the local and national level to support primary and secondary prevention strategies. The Stop It Now! Helpline is a toll-free number for adults who are at risk for sexually abusing a child, for friends and family members of sexual abusers and/or victims, and for parents of children with sexual behavior problems. All calls are confidential and will be answered by a trained staff member.

  351 Pleasant Street, Suite B319
  Northampton, MA 01060
  Help line: (888) PREVENT (888-773-8368)
  (413) 587-3500
  Fax: (413) 587-3505
  Email: info@stopitnow.com
  www.stopitnow.com

Survivorship

For survivors of ritualistic abuse, mind control, and torture.

  3181 Mission Street, #139
  San Francisco, CA 94110
  www.survivorship.org

Survivors Network of Those Abused By Priests (SNAP)

The Survivors Network of Those Abused by Priests (SNAP) is a self-help organization of adult survivors of clergy sexual abuse and their supporters. They work to end the cycle of abuse in two ways: by supporting one another in personal healing and by pursuing justice and institutional change by holding individual perpetrators responsible and the church accountable. SNAP has local chapters and support groups in over fifty cities across the country. Via their Web site, SNAP provides resources such as peer counseling, contact information for local support groups, online discussion boards, and a library of educational materials and news stories and ways to support their mission, both in the local community and on a national level. The SNAP Web site includes contact information for local SNAP chapters.

  P.O. Box 6416
  Chicago, IL 60680-6416
  Toll-free: (877) SNAPHEALS
  (877-762-7432)
  Email: SNAPBlaine@hotmail.com
  www.snapnetwork.org

Childhood Sexual Abuse (cont.)

WEB SITES (cont.)

Survivors of Incest Anonymous (SIA)
SIA World Service Office serves the many independent SIA support groups around the world, as well as individuals who contact them. SIA also publishes and sells incest survivor–related literature, maintains a directory of meetings, and publishes a quarterly bulletin. An individual can send a self-addressed envelope and $3.00 (if possible) or call the SIA information line to request a directory of meetings. One can also contact SIA to ask questions or to obtain literature.

    World Service Office, P.O. Box 190
    Benson, MD 21018-9998
    (410) 893-3322
    www.siawso.org

VOICES In Action, Inc.
VIA is an international nonprofit organization providing support for victims of incest and child sexual abuse. VIA helps victims of incest and child sexual abuse to become survivors and generates public awareness of the prevalence of incest, its impact, and how it can be prevented or stopped through educational programs. VIA also serves as a clearinghouse and dissemination center connecting victims and survivors to local resources.

    Email: voicesinaction@aol.com

General Trauma

Attachment, Trauma, and Healing: Understanding and Treating Attachment Disorder in Children and Families by Terry M. Levy and Michael Orlans (CWLA/Child Welfare League of America Press, 1998).

Post-Traumatic Stress Disorder Sourcebook by Glenn R. Schiraldi (McGraw-Hill, 2000).

Trauma and Recovery: The Aftermath of Violence From Domestic Abuse to Political Terror by Judith Lewis Herman, MD (Basic Books, 1993).

Unchained Memories: True Stories of Traumatic Memories, Lost and Found by Lenore Terr (Basic Books, 1994).

Social Trauma

The Assault on Truth: Freud's Suppression of the Seduction Theory by Geoffrey Masson (Farrar, Straus and Giroux, 1984).

The Body in Pain: The Making and Unmaking of the World by Elaine Scarry (Oxford University Press, 1986).

Boys Will Be Boys: Breaking the Link Between Masculinity and Violence by Myriam Miedzian (Lantern Books, 2002).

The Chalice and the Blade: Our History, Our Future by Riane Eisler (Harper San Francisco, 1988).

The Feast of the Goat: A Novel by Mario Vargas Llosa (Picador USA, 2002).

Home Front: Notes from the Family War Zone by Louise Armstrong (McGraw-Hill, 1984).

Homophobia: How We All Pay the Price edited by Warren J. Blumenfeld (Beacon Press, 1992).

A Human Being Died That Night: A South African Story of Forgiveness by Pumla Gobodo-Madikizela (Mariner Books, 2004).

Medicine Stories: History, Culture, and the Politics of Integrity by Aurora Levins Morales (South End Press, 1998).

Methodology of the Oppressed by Chela Sandoval (University of Minnesota Press, 2000).

Native American Postcolonial Psychology by Bonnie and Eduardo Duran (CUNY Press, 1995). This book deals with the consequences of trauma on historically oppressed people. These authors are responsible for creating a new theory and practice within psychology around understanding the impacts of colonialism and healing from them in a way that challenges and transforms oppression and oppressive relationships.

One Nation, Underprivileged: Why American Poverty Affects Us All by Mark Robert Rank (Oxford University Press, 2004).

We Wish to Inform You That Tomorrow We Will be Killed With Our Families: Stories from Rwanda by Philip Gourevitch (Picador, 1999).

Whitewashing Race: The Myth of a Color-Blind Society edited by Michael K. Brown (University of California Press, 2003).

Trauma, the Brain, And Memory

EMDR: The Breakthrough Therapy for Overcoming Anxiety, Stress, and Trauma by Francine Shapiro and Margot Silk Forrest (HarperCollins, 1997).

Genome: The Autobiography of a Species in 23 Chapters by Matt Ridley (HarperCollins, 2000).

Mind Wide Open: Your Brain and the Neuro-Science of Everyday Life by Steven Johnson (Scribner, 2004).

Why Zebras Don't Get Ulcers, 3rd edition, by Robert M. Sapolsky (Owl Books, 2004).

Trauma in Film

Amandla! A Revolution in Four-Part Harmony (2002)

Boys Don't Cry (1999)

Monster (2003)

Murder on a Sunday Morning (2001)

Once Were Warriors (1995)

Rabbit-Proof Fence (2002)

The Woodsman (2004)

Trauma in Literature

Bastard Out of Carolina by Dorothy Allison (Plume, 1993).

Ceremony by Leslie Marmon Silko (Penguin Books, 1977).

The Color Purple by Alice Walker (Harvest, 2003).

The Feast of the Goat: A Novel by Mario Vargas Llosa (Picador USA, 2002).

The Kite Runner by Khaled Hosseini (Riverhead Trade, 2004).

Mysterious Skin: A Novel by Scott Heim (Perennial, 1996).

Not Vanishing by Chrystos (Press Gang Publishers, 1989).

Trauma and Recovery Resources

WEB SITES

Institute on Violence, Abuse, and Trauma
An excellent networking, education, and training clearinghouse.
6160 Cornerstone Court East
San Diego, CA 92121
(858) 623-2777
www.ivatcenters.org

International Trauma-Healing Institute
Nonprofit organization dedicated to global trauma healing.
269 S. Lorraine Blvd.
Los Angeles, CA 90004
(323) 954-1400
www.traumainstitute.org
info@traumainstitute.org

Trauma and Recovery Resources (cont.)

WEB SITES (cont.)

Trauma Information Pages, David Baldwin

These Trauma Pages focus primarily on emotional trauma and traumatic stress, including PTSD (post-traumatic stress disorder) and dissociation, whether following individual traumatic experience(s) or a large-scale disaster. The purpose of this site is to provide information for clinicians and researchers in the traumatic stress field, including what goes on biologically in the brain during traumatic experience and its healing.

    www.trauma-pages.com

The Wounded Healer Journal (TWHJ)

TWHJ is an Internet pioneer in the area of online support for trauma and abuse survivors. This virtual community journal offers an array of Web services for those who have experienced the devastation of traumatic experiences, including child abuse. TWHJ provides links to national therapists, crisis numbers, support chat rooms, and a Web store. It offers similar services for partners and allies of sexual assault survivors. Linda Chapman is the creator, editor, and administrator of TWHJ.

    Email: Linda_twhj@yahoo.com
    www.twhj.com

HARMFUL SUBSTANCE USE AND RECOVERY

Al-Anon Family Groups

Twelve-Step program modeled on Alcoholics Anonymous for people in close relationships with those who use alcohol in a way that harms themselves and others.

    1600 Corporate Landing Parkway
    Virginia Beach, VA 23454
    (757) 563-1600
    www.al-anon.org

Alcoholics Anonymous

Twelve-Step program for people who use alcohol in a way that harms themselves and others.

    P.O. Box 459
    New York, NY 10163
    (212) 870-3400
    www.alcoholics-anonymous.org

Debtors Anonymous

Twelve-Step program modeled on Alcoholics Anonymous for people who use debting or spending (money, time, or love) in a way that harms themselves and others.

    P.O. Box 920888
    Needham, MA 02492
    (781) 453-2743
    www.debtorsanonymous.org

Trauma and Recovery Resources (cont.)

HARMFUL SUBSTANCE USE
AND RECOVERY (cont.)

Harm Reduction Coalition
The Harm Reduction Coalition is a national advocacy and capacity-building organization that promotes the health and dignity of individuals and communities impacted by drug use. HRC advances policies and programs that help people address the adverse effects of drug use including overdose, HIV, hepatitis C, addiction, and incarceration. We recognize that the structures of social inequality impact the lives and options of affected communities differently, and work to uphold individuals' rights to health and well-being, as well as in their competence to protect themselves, their loved ones, and their communities.
22 West 27th Street, 5th Floor
New York, NY 10001
(212) 213-6376
1440 Broadway, Suite 510
Oakland, CA 94612
(510) 444-6969
www.harmreduction.org

Narcotics Anonymous
Twelve-Step program modeled on Alcoholics Anonymous for people who use prescription or street drugs in a way that harms themselves and others.
P.O. Box 9999
Van Nuys, CA 91409
(818) 773-9999
www.na.org

Overeaters Anonymous
Twelve-Step program modeled on Alcoholics Anonymous for people who use food in a way that harms themselves and others.
P.O. Box 44020
Rio Rancho, NM 87174
(505) 891-2664
www.overeatersanonymous.org

Sex and Love Addicts Anonymous
Twelve-Step program modeled on Alcoholics Anonymous for people who use sex or relationships in a way that harms themselves and others.
1550 NE Loop 410, Suite 118
San Antonio, TX 78209
(210) 828-7900
www.slaafws.org

Women for Sobriety
P.O. Box 618
Quakertown, PA 18951
(215) 536-8026
www.womenforsobriety.org

SOMATIC HEALING

BOOKS

The Anatomy of Change: A Way to Move Through Life's Transitions by Richard Strozzi-Heckler (North Atlantic Books, 1993).

Being Human at Work edited by Richard Strozzi-Heckler (North Atlantic Books, 2003).

Bioenergetics by Alexander Lowen (Penguin, 1994).

Body-Centered Psychotherapy: The Hakomi Method: The Integrated Use of Mindfulness, Nonviolence, and the Body by Ron Kurtz (Life Rhythm, 1990).

The Body in Psychotherapy: Inquiries in Somatic Psychology (Body in Psychotherapy, Vol. 3) by Don Hanlon Johnson (North Atlantic Books, 1998).

The Body in Recovery: Somatic Psychotherapy and the Self by John P. Conger (Frog Ltd., 1994).

The Body Remembers: The Psychophysiology of Trauma and Trauma Treatment by Babette Rothschild (W.W. Norton and Company, 2000).

Bone, Breath, and Gesture: Practices of Embodiment by Don Hanlon Johnson (North Atlantic Books, 1995).

Emotional Anatomy: The Structure of Experience by Stanley Keleman (Center Press, 1986).

Getting in Touch: A Guide to New Body-Centered Therapies by Christine Caldwell (Quest Books, 1997).

Getting Our Bodies Back by Christine Caldwell (Shambhala, 1996).

Healing Sex: The Complete Guide to Sexual Wholeness by Staci Haines (DVD by SIR Productions, 2004).

Holding the Center: Sanctuary in a Time of Confusion by Richard Strozzi-Heckler (Frog, Ltd., 1997).

The Intuitive Body: Aikido as a Clairsentient Practice by Wendy Palmer (North Atlantic Books, 1994).

The Life We Are Given: A Long-Term Program for Realizing the Potential of Body, Mind, Heart, and Soul by George Leonard and Michael Murphy (Jeremy P. Tarcher, 1995).

Somatics: Reawakening the Mind's Control of Movement, Flexibility, and Health by Thomas Hanna (HarperCollins Publishers, 1988).

Healing Sex: A Mind–Body Approach to Healing Sexual Trauma by Staci Haines (Cleis Press, 2007).

Victims of Cruelty: Somatic Psychotherapy in the Treatment of Posttraumatic Stress Disorder by Marianna Eckberg (North Atlantic Books, 2000).

Waking the Tiger: Healing Trauma: The Innate Capacity to Transform Overwhelming Experiences by Peter A. Levine and Ann Frederick (North Atlantic Books, 1997).

Your Body Speaks Its Mind by Stanley Keleman (Center Press, 1981).

Somatic Healing (cont.)

WEB SITES

Generative Somatics—Staci Haines

Generative Somatics is an integrative approach using somatic awareness, somatic bodywork, and somatic practices to create lasting change. Generative Somatics approaches trauma as both an individual and a collective experience. In this work we address individual experiences of trauma and the social context in which we are living to understand, heal, and transform. Generative Somatics is used in one-on-one and group work as well as in social change and community-building settings.

www.somaticsandtrauma.org

Healing Sex, DVD

This DVD describes the Generative Somatics approach to healing intimacy, relationship, and sexuality after sexual trauma. A diverse cast demonstrates the healing process including somatic embodiment, somatic bodywork, and somatic practices. By Staci Haines and SIR Productions.

www.healingsexthemovie.com

Rubenfeld Synergy Method

The Rubenfeld Synergy Method is a holistic therapy that integrates body, mind, spirit, and emotions. Developed by Ilana Rubenfeld in the 1960s, Rubenfeld Synergy uses gentle touch, along with verbal dialogue, active listening, Gestalt Process, imagery, metaphor, movement, and humor to invite the body into the healing process.

www.rubenfeldsynergy.com

Sensorimotor Psychotherapy Institute—Pat Ogden

The Sensorimotor Psychotherapy Institute (SPI) is an educational organization dedicated to the study and teaching of a body-oriented approach to clinical psychotherapy practice.

www.sensorimotorpsychotherapy.org

Somatic Experiencing and The Foundation for Human Enrichment—Peter Levine

The Foundation for Human Enrichment (FHE) provides individuals, families, and communities with effective "self-help" tools for healing trauma. We recognize the relationship between trauma and the igniting of violence and war. Our goal is to help end this destructive cycle. Links and Resources.

www.traumahealing.com

Strozzi Institute—Richard Strozzi-Heckler

Strozzi Institute is the premier training institute for Embodied Leadership. For more than thirty years, Strozzi Institute has provided an innovative learning environment using somatics to develop leadership, create organizational change, and encourage social vision. The institute offers public and private programs for corporations, small businesses, and individuals interested in developing their leadership presence and effectiveness. In addition, it offers a unique coaching certification program that teaches the relevance of the body in coaching.

www.strozziinstitute.com

The Trauma Center

Contains numerous articles by Bessel van der Kolk and other trauma-related publications. This is a great resource for the latest studies on brain development, psychobiology, and trauma.

www.traumacenter.org

SEX-POSITIVE BOOKS AND RESOURCES

Sex Guides

All About Birth Control: The Complete Guide by Planned Parenthood (Three Rivers Press/Crown, 1998).

Anal Pleasure and Health by Jack Morin, PhD. (Down There Press, 1998).

The Erotic Mind: Unlocking the Inner Sources of Sexual Passion and Fulfillment by Jack Morin, PhD. (HarperCollins, 1996). A guide to increasing and enhancing arousal.

The Ethical Slut: A Guide to Infinite Sexual Possibilities by Dossie Easton and Catherine Liszt (Greenery Press, 1998). Information and advice about responsible nonmonogamy and polyamory.

Exhibitionism for the Shy by Carol Queen (Down There Press, 1995). Advice on communicating sexual desires.

The Fine Art of Erotic Talk: How to Entice, Excite, and Enchant Your Lover With Words by Bonnie Gabriel (Bantam, 1996). Tips on erotic talk and sexual communication.

The Good Vibrations Guide to Sex: The Most Complete Sex Manual Ever by Cathy Winks and Anne Semans (Cleis Press, 2002). A comprehensive manual covering all aspects of female and male sexuality; extensive resource section.

The Guide to Getting It On by Paul Joannides (Goofy Foot Press, 2006). Humorous heterosexual guide with detailed advice about sexual technique and communication.

Sexual Pleasure: Reaching New Heights of Sexual Arousal and Intimacy by Barbara Keesling, PhD. (Hunter House, 2004). Focuses on creating sexual intimacy.

Turn Ons: Pleasing Yourself While You Please Your Lover by Lonnie Barbach, PhD. (Plume, 1998). A guide to enhancing sexual communication and creativity.

The Ultimate Guide to Sex and Disability: For All of Us Who Live with Disabilities, Chronic Pain, and Illness by Miriam Kaufman, MD, Cory Silverberg, and Fran Odette (Cleis Press, 2007).

Sex Guides (cont.)

CHILDREN AND TEENS

All About Sex: A Family Resource on Sex and Sexuality by Planned Parenthood (Three Rivers Press/Crown, 1997). A reference on sex and sexual health.

Changing Bodies, Changing Lives: A Book for Teens on Sex and Relationships by Ruth Bell (Three Rivers Press, 1988). A thorough, inclusive guide.

The First Time: What Parents and Teenage Girls Should Know About Losing Your Virginity by Karen Bouris (Conari Press, 1995). Firsthand accounts from a number of women, with both positive and negative perceptions.

How Sex Works by Elizabeth Fenwick and Richard Walker (Dorling Kindersley, 1994). Advice and information for teens.

It's Perfectly Normal: Changing Bodies, Growing Up, Sex, and Sexual Health by Robie H. Harris (Candlewick Press, 2004). Information on sexual health and self-esteem for kids ages seven to fourteen.

Just Say Yes/Di que si by The Coalition for Positive Sexuality (The Coalition for Positive Sexuality, 1998). Explicit advice on AIDS, STDs, pregnancy, homosexuality, and self-esteem for teens. In English or Spanish.

A Kid's First Book About Sex by Joani Blank (Down There Press, 1993). Information for kids ages seven and up.

La Menstruacion by Joann Gardner-Loulan, Bonnie Lopez, and Marcia Quackenbush (Parramon, 1993). Spanish-language version of *Period*, a guide to menstruation for adolescent girls.

Period by Joann Gardner-Loulan, Bonnie Lopez, and Marcia Quackenbush (Volcano Press, 1991). Guide to menstruation for adolescent girls.

The Period Book: Everything You Don't Want to Ask (But Need to Know) by Karen and Jennifer Gravelle (Walker Books for Young Readers, 2006). A guide for girls about the physical, emotional, and social changes that accompany puberty. Also available in Spanish, *El libro del periodo* (Walker, 2003).

Talking With Your Child About Sex: Questions and Answers for Children From Birth to Puberty by Dr. Mary Calderone and Dr. James Ramey (Ballantine Books, 1983). Examples of children's sex questions with suggested answers.

What's Happening to My Body? A Book for Boys by Lynda Madaras (Newmarket Press, 2007). For adolescents and their parents.

What's Happening to My Body? A Book for Girls by Lynda Madaras (Newmarket Press, 2007). For adolescents and their parents.

Sex Guides (cont.)

EASTERN APPROACHES TO SEXUALITY

Acupressure for Lovers: Secrets of Touch for Increasing Intimacy by Michael Reed Gach, PhD. (Bantam Doubleday Dell, 1997). Combines Eastern and Western techniques.

The Illustrated Kama Sutra translated by Sir Richard Burton (Standard Publications, 2004). Excerpts from the classic Indian love texts, with illustrations.

The Multi-Orgasmic Couple: Sexual Secrets Every Couple Should Know by Mantak Chia (HarperOne, 2002).

Passion Play: Ancient Secrets for a Lifetime of Health and Happiness Through Sensational Sex by Felice Dunas, PhD., with Philip Goldberg (Riverhead Books, 1998). Holistic guidance on sexual healing, seduction, and harnessing Chi energy.

Sacred Sex by Jwala (Mandala, 1993). An illustrated guide to Tantric sex.

Tantra: A Guide to Conscious Loving by Charles Muir and Caroline Muir (Mercury House, 1989). Teaches heterosexual couples to increase intimacy using sexual energy.

Tantric Sex for Women: A Guide for Lesbian, Bi, Hetero, and Solo Lovers by Christa Schulte (Hunter House, 2005). Exceptional manual for enhancing the sexual and spiritual life of women using Tantric principles.

The Tao of Sexual Massage: A Step-by-Step Guide to Exciting, Enduring, Loving Pleasure by Stephen Russell (Fireside, 2003). Sexual massage techniques using Taoist concepts of energy.

MASTURBATION

First Person Sexual edited by Joani Blank (Down There Press, 1996). An anthology of firsthand masturbation accounts from women and men.

For Yourself: The Fulfillment of Female Sexuality by Lonnie Barbach, PhD. (Signet/ Penguin, 2000). A guide for women seeking to enhance their sexual experience; aimed at women who have never had an orgasm.

I Am My Lover: Women Pleasure Themselves edited by Joani Blank (Down There Press, 1997). Photos and essays about female masturbation.

The Joy of Solo Sex by Dr. Harold Litten (Factor Press, 1993). Teaches masturbation techniques and sex-positivity for men.

Sex For One: The Joy of Self-Loving by Betty Dodson (Three Rivers Press/Crown, 1996). Teaches masturbation techniques and sex-positivity for women.

Solitary Sex: A Cultural History of Masturbation by Thomas W. Laqueur (Zone Books, 2004).

Tickle Your Fancy: A Woman's Guide to Self-Pleasure by Sadie Allison (Tickle Kitty Press, 2001).

Sex Guides (cont.)

MEN'S SEXUALITY

Great Sex: A Man's Guide to the Secret Principles of Total-Body Sex by Michael Castleman (Rodale Press, 2004).

Men in Love by Nancy Friday (Arrow, 2003). A collection of men's sexual fantasies.

Men Loving Men: A Gay Sex Guide and Consciousness Book by Mitch Walker (Gay Sunshine Press, 1997). A guide to all aspects of gay male sexuality.

The Multi-Orgasmic Man: How Any Man Can Experience Multiple Orgasms and Dramatically Enhance His Sexual Relationship by Mantak Chia and Douglas Abrams Arava (HarperSanFrancisco, 1996). Incorporates Eastern and Western sexual techniques.

Sexual Solutions: A Guide for Men and the Women Who Love Them by Michael Castleman (Simon and Schuster, 1989). A thorough sex manual that includes a chapter for men whose partners have been raped.

POLITICS AND PRO-SEX FEMINISM

Annie Sprinkle: Post Porn Modernist: My Twenty-Five Years as a Multimedia Whore by Annie Sprinkle (Cleis Press, 1998). Autobiography, cultural history, spiritual journey, and political memoir by a sex worker and cult star.

Caught Looking: Feminism, Pornography, and Censorship by the FACT Book Committee (Long River Books, 1988). Essays and photography exploring sexual expression and censorship.

Global Sex Workers: Rights, Resistance, and Redefinition edited by Kamala Kempadoo and Jo Doezema (Routledge, 1998). Essays and studies about prostitution around the world, offering new perspectives on sex work's possibilities for empowerment and exploitation.

My Gender Workbook by Kate Bornstein (Routledge, 1998). A guidebook encouraging an exploration of personal and cultural assumptions about gender.

Real Live Nude Girl: Chronicles of Sex-Positive Culture by Carol Queen (Cleis Press, 1997). Essays by author, sexologist, and self-proclaimed exhibitionist Carol Queen.

Sex Changes: The Politics of Transgenderism by Patrick Califia (Cleis Press, 2003). An analysis of the contemporary history of transsexuality.

Sex Work: Writings by Women in the Sex Industry edited by Frédérique Delacoste (Cleis Press, 1998). Writings by a diverse group of sex workers.

Sex Guides (cont.)

RELATIONSHIPS

Conscious Loving: The Journey to Co-Commitment by Gay Hendricks, PhD., and Kathlyn Hendricks, PhD. (Bantam Books, 1990).

Getting the Love You Want by Harville Hendrix, PhD. (Pocket Books, 2005).

Hot Monogamy: Essential Steps to More Passionate, Intimate Lovemaking by Dr. Patricia Love and Jo Robinson (Plume/Penguin, 1994). Advice and information for monogamous couples.

Lesbian Couples: A Guide to Creating Healthy Relationships by D. Merilee Clunis and G. Dorsey Green (Seal Press, 2004).

The Lesbian and Gay Book of Love and Marriage: Creating the Stories of Our Lives by Paula Martinac (Broadway Books, 1998).

The Passionate Marriage: Sex, Love, and Intimacy in Emotionally Committed Relationships by David Schnarch, PhD. (W.W. Norton and Co., 1997).

S/M AND POWER PLAY

Different Loving: The World of Sexual Dominance and Submission by Gloria G. Brame, William D. Brame, and Jon Jacobs (Villard/Random Books, 1995).

Learning the Ropes: A Basic Guide to Safe and Fun S/M Lovemaking by Race Bannon (Daedalus Publishing Co., 1992).

The New Bottoming Book by Dossie Easton and Janet Hardy (Greenery Press, 2001).

The New Topping Book by Dossie Easton and Janet Hardy (Greenery Press, 2001).

Sensuous Magic: A Guide to S/M for Adventurous Couples by Patrick Califia (Cleis Press, 2002).

The Sexually Dominant Woman: A Workbook for Nervous Beginners by Lady Green (Greenery Press, 1998).

SM 101: A Realistic Introduction by Jay Wiseman (Greenery Press, 1998). Instruction and resource listings.

Sex Guides (cont.)

WOMEN'S SEXUALITY

Are We Having Fun Yet? The Intelligent Woman's Guide to Sex by Marcia Douglass, PhD., and Lisa Douglass, PhD. (Hyperion, 1997).

Becoming Orgasmic: A Sexual and Personal Growth Program for Women by Julia R. Heiman, PhD., and Joseph Lopiccolo, PhD. (Fireside/Simon and Schuster, 1988).

The Black Women's Health Book edited by Evelyn C. White (Seal Press, 1994).

The Erotic Lives of Women edited by Linda Troeller (Scallo, 1998).

Femalia edited by Joani Blank (Down There Press, 1993).

I Love Female Orgasm: An Extraordinary Orgasm Guide by Dorian Solot and Marshall Miller (Marlowe and Co., 2007).

In the Garden of Desire: Women's Sexual Fantasies as a Gateway to Passion and Pleasure by Wendy Maltz and Suzie Boss (Broadway/Bantam Doubleday Dell, 1997).

The Multi-Orgasmic Woman: Discover Your Full Desire, Pleasure, and Vitality by Mantak Chia (Rodale Books, 2006).

My Secret Garden by Nancy Friday (Simon and Schuster, 1998).

The New Ourselves, Growing Older: Women Aging with Knowledge and Power by Paula B. Doress-Worters and Diana Laskin Siegal (Touchstone/Simon and Schuster, 1994).

A New View of a Woman's Body by the Federation of Feminist Women's Health Centers (Feminist Health Press, 1995).

Our Bodies, Ourselves: A New Edition for a New Era by the Boston Women's Health Book Collective (Touchstone, 2005).

Our Bodies, Ourselves: Menopause by the Boston Women's Health Book Collective (Touchstone, 2006).

The Sexuality of Latinas edited by Norma Alarcón, Ana Castillo, and Cherríe Moraga (Third Woman Press, 1993).

Smart Girls Guide to the G-Spot by Violet Blue (Cleis Press, 2007).

The Ultimate Guide to Anal Sex for Women by Tristan Taormino (Cleis Press, 2006).

The Ultimate Guide to Cunnilingus by Violet Blue (Cleis Press, 2002).

The Whole Lesbian Sex Book: A Passionate Guide for All of Us by Felice Newman (Cleis Press, 2004).

A Woman's Guide to Overcoming Sexual Fear and Pain by Aurelie Jones Goodwin, EdD, and Marc E. Agronin, MD (New Harbinger Publications, 1997).

Sex Guides (cont.)

SAFER SEX RESOURCES

American Social Health Association
STI Resource Center Hotline
(800) 227-8922
www.ashastd.org

Boston Women's Health Book Collective
(617) 451-3666
www.ourbodiesourselves.org

Centers for Disease Control
(404) 639-3534
www.cdc.gov

   HIV/AIDS
   (800) 232-4636
   www.cdc.gov/hiv

   National Prevention Information Network
   (800) 458-5231
   www.cdcnpin.org/scripts/index.asp

LesbianSTD.com
(206) 731-3679
depts.washington.edu/wswstd

Planned Parenthood
(800) 230-PLAN
www.ppfa.org

Sex Education and Information Resources

The Body Electric School
Teaches people to experience their potential
as healers of self and others through touch,
conscious breath, and honoring the wisdom
of the body.
   6527A Telegraph Avenue
   Oakland, CA 94609
   (510) 653-1594
   www.bodyelectric.org

Center for Sex and Culture
Provides nonjudgmental, sex-positive sexuality education and support to diverse populations through classes, social gatherings,
hands-on, practical skills-building events,
research, and a library of sex-positive information. Their mission is to effect sex-positive
cultural change. Founded by Carol Queen
and Robert Lawrence.
   www.sexandculture.org

Coalition for Positive Sexuality
A fantastic resource for teens with any questions about sex. Includes plenty of information on safer sex and contraception (in
English and Spanish), along with a discussion
board.
   P.O. Box 77212
   Washington, DC 20013
   www.positive.org

Human Awareness Institute
An organization that produces workshops on
love, intimacy, and sexuality.
   700 Widgeon St.
   Foster City, CA 94404-1336
   (800) 800-4117
   www.hai.org

Institute for the Advanced Study of Human Sexuality (IASHS)
School with a postgraduate degree program in
human sexuality studies. IASHS also produces educational pamphlets, books, videos,
and safer sex supply kits.
   1523 Franklin Street
   San Francisco, CA 94109
   (415) 928-1133
   www.iashs.edu

Kink Aware Professionals
Service offered by the National Coalition for
Sexual Freedom providing referrals to psychotherapeutic, medical, and legal professionals who are knowledgeable about and
sensitive to diverse expressions of sexuality.
   www.ncsfreedom.org/kap/

The Kinsey Institute for Research in Sex, Gender, and Reproduction
The mission of the Kinsey Institute is to pro-
mote interdisciplinary research and scholar-
ship in the fields of human sexuality, gender,
and reproduction.
   Morrison 313, Indiana University
   Bloomington, IN 47405
   (812) 855-7686
   www.indiana.edu/~kinsey

Queernet.org
QueerNet provides dozens of email discussion
lists for the gay, lesbian, bisexual, transgendered, and S/M communities. The Web site
gives detailed information on how to sub-
scribe to the lists, which include many supportive lists for women exploring all facets of
sexuality and gender.
   www.queernet.org

Sex Education and Information Resources (cont.)

San Francisco Sex Information
Free information and referral switchboard
providing anonymous, accurate, nonjudgmental information about sex.
   (415) 989-7374
   www.sfsi.org

Sexual Health Network
A terrific resource addressing the sexual concerns of those with disabilities, injuries, and
illnesses.
   www.sexualhealth.com

**Sexuality Information and Education
Council of the U.S. (SIECUS)**
A national, nonprofit advocacy organization
that develops, collects, and disseminates
information; promotes comprehensive education about sexuality; and advocates the rights
of individuals to make responsible sexual
choices.
   130 W. 42nd Street, Suite 350
   New York, NY 10036
   (212) 819-9770
   www.siecus.org

Society for Human Sexuality
A comprehensive online library of sexuality
resources.
   www.sexuality.org

**The Society for the Scientific Study of
Sexuality (SSSS)**
An international organization dedicated to
the advancement of knowledge about sexuality.
   P.O. Box 416
   Allentown, PA 18105
   (610) 530-2483
   www.sexscience.org

SEX TOY STORES AND
MAIL ORDER RESOURCES

The following stores and online catalogs are a great place to find the latest in sex education, books, DVDs, and toys.

Adam and Eve
(800) 293-4654
www.aeonline.com

Babeland
(800) 658-9119
www.babeland.com

7007 Melrose Avenue
Los Angeles, CA 90038
(323) 634-9480

707 E. Pike Street
Seattle, WA 98122
(206) 328-2914

94 Rivington Street
New York City, NY 10002
(212) 375-1701

43 Mercer Street
New York, NY 10013
(212) 966-2120

Blowfish
(800) 325-2569
www.blowfish.com

Come As You Are
Web site features resources on sex and disability.
701 Queen Street West
Toronto, ON M6J 1E6 Canada
(877) 858.3160
www.comeasyouare.com

Condomania
(800) 926-6366
www.condomania.com

Eve's Garden
119 W. 57th Street, 12th Floor
New York, NY 10019
(800) 848-3837
www.evesgarden.com

Fatale Media
Explicit DVDs "for lesbians and other sexually adventurous souls."
www.fatalemedia.com

Forbidden Fruit
Fetish boutique.
512 Neches
Austin, TX 78701
(512) 487-8358
(800) 315-2029
www.forbiddenfruit.com

Good Vibrations
(800) 289-8423
www.goodvibes.com

308-A Harvard Street
Brookline, MA 02446
(617) 264-4400

603 Valencia Street
San Francisco, CA 94110
(415) 522-5460

1620 Polk Street
San Francisco, CA 94109
(415) 345-0400

2504 San Pablo Avenue
Berkeley, CA 94702
(510) 841-8987

Smitten Kitten
3010 Lyndale Avenue South
Minneapolis, MN 55408
(888) 751-0523
www.smittenkittenonline.com

Stormy Leather
Leather and fetish wear.
1158 Howard Street
San Francisco, CA 94103
(415) 626-1672
(800) 486-9650
www.stormyleather.com

A Woman's Touch
600 Williamson Street
Madison, WI 53703
888-621-8880
www.a-womans-touch.com

Womyn's Ware
896 Commercial Drive
Vancouver, BC V5L 3Y5 Canada
(888) 996-9273
www.womynsware.com

Xandria Collection
(800) 242-2823
www.xandria.com

About the Author

STACI HAINES is the author of *Healing Sex: A Mind-Body Approach to Healing Sexual Trauma*, originally published as *The Survivor's Guide to Sex* (Cleis Press, 1999, 2007), and the DVD *Healing Sex* (SIR Productions, 2005), both offering a mind/body (somatic) approach to healing from sexual trauma and developing vital sexual and intimate relationships. She is the originator of the Generative Somatics approach, specializing in healing trauma, and leads courses teaching this work to community activists, social leaders, therapists, and other practitioners. Haines is the founder of generation FIVE, a national nonprofit whose mission is to end the sexual abuse of children within five generations. She has been organizing and educating in the area of child sexual abuse since 1985 and has been a trained sex educator since 1991. She is a longtime activist in the areas of sexual assault, racial justice, and environmental sustainability. Staci is committed to combining personal healing and social justice work, and sees that both need to be addressed to bring about life affirming change in the world.

Made in United States
Troutdale, OR
02/27/2025

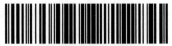

29365281R00178